Micronutrient Testing

How To Find What Vitamins, Minerals, and Antioxidants You Need

Dr. Kelly Miller, DC, NMD, FASA, FBAARM, CFMP

Micronutrient Testing: How To Find What Vitamins, Minerals, and Antioxidants You Need

Book 2 of the *Health Restoration Series*
      Series Editor, George Ann Gregory, Ph.D.

Second Edition
Copyright © 2017 Kelly Miller

Some content in this book has been adapted from SpectraCell Laboratories, Inc.

Printed by CreateSpace, An Amazon.com Company
CreateSpace, Charleston, SC

ISBN 13: 978-0-9979113-5-0
ISBN 10: 0-9979113-5-2

Dedication

I dedicate this book to all the people who are seeking information about how to better meet their nutritional needs.

Acknowledgements

I could not have written this book without the support and encouragement of my best friend and soul mate, Dr. Debra Hoffman. I would like to give a special thanks to Spectracell Laboratory for giving me liberal use of their information in printed format and from the Internet. I give thanks to my sister, Dr. George Ann Gregory for her editing, Emz Wright for the book cover, and Deepali Gupta for the one illustration.

I have been guided by the following Biblical passages.

Proverbs 8:1-36, 9:1

Does wisdom not cry out, and understand lift up her voice? She takes her stand on the top of the high hill, beside the way, where the paths meet. She cries out by the gates, at the entry of the city, at the entrance of the doors: "To you, O men, I call, and my voice is to the sons of men. O you simple ones, understand prudence, and you fools, be of understanding heart. Listen, for I will speak of excellent things, and from the opening of my lips, will come right things. For my mouth will speak truth: wickedness is an abomination to my lips. All the words of my mouth are with righteousness; nothing crooked or perverse is in them. They are all plain to him that understands, and right to those who find knowledge. Receive my instruction, and not silver, and knowledge rather than choice gold; For wisdom is better than rubies, and all the things one may desire cannot be compared to her. "I, wisdom, dwell with prudence, and find out knowledge and discretion. The fear of the Lord is to hate evil; pride and arrogance and the evil way and perverse mouth I hate. Counsel is mine, and sound wisdom; I am understanding, I have strength. By me kings reign, and rulers decree justice. By me princes rule, and nobles, all the judges of the earth. I love those who love me, and those who seek me diligently will find me. Riches and honor are with me, enduring riches and righteousness. My fruit is better than gold, yes, than fine gold, and my revenue than fine silver. I transverse the way of righteousness, in the midst of justice, That I may cause those who love me to inherit wealth, that I may fill their treasures. "The Lord possessed me, at the beginning of His way, before His works of old. I have been established from everylasting. From the beginning, before there was an earth. When there was no depth I was brought forth, when there were no fountains abounding

---

with water. Before the mountains were settled, before the hills, I was brought forth; while as yet He had not made the earth or the fields, or the primal dust of the world. When He prepared the heavens, I was there, when He drew a circle on the face of the deep, When He established clouds above, when He strengthened the fountains of the deep, When He assigned to the sea its limit, so that the waters would not transgress His command, when He marked out the foundations of the earth, Then I was beside Him as a master craftsman; and I was daily His delight, rejoicing always before Him, Rejoicing in His inhabited world, and my delight was with the sons of men. "Now therefore, listen to me my children, for blessed are those who keep my ways. Hear instruction and be wise, and do not disdain it. Blessed is the man who listens to me, watching daily at my gates, waiting at the posts of my doors. For whoever finds me finds life, and obtains favor from the Lord; But he who sins against me wrongs his own soul; all those who hate me love death." Wisdom has built her house, she has hewn out her seven pillars. *NKJV*

Proverbs 9:9-11
Give instruction to a wise man, he will be yet wiser: teach a just man, and he will increase in learning. For the fear of the Lord is the beginning of wisdom; and the knowledge of the holy is understanding. For by me thy days shall be multiplied and the years of thy life shall be increased. *NKJV*

James: 13-17
Who is wise and understanding among you? Let him show by good conduct that his works are done in the meekness of wisdom. But if you have bitter envy and self-seeking in your hearts, do not trust and lie against the truth. This wisdom does not descend from above, but is earthly, sensual, demonic. For where envy and self-seeking exist, confusion and every evil thing are there. But the wisdom that is from above is first pure, then peaceable, gentle, willing to yield, full of mercy and good fruits, without partiality and without hypocrisy. *NKJV*

Disclaimer

This publication is designed to provide scientific, authoritative, and personal anecdotal information in regard to the subject matter covered. The reader understands that the author is not engaged in rendering professional services. If you require medical, psychological, or any other expert assistance, please seek the services of a professional.

The information, personal experiences, anecdotal stories, procedures, and suggestions contained in the book are not intended to replace the services of a trained health-care professional or to serve as a replacement for a health-care professional's advice and care. You should consult a health-care professional regarding any of this information, ideas, personal experiences, anecdotal stories, procedures, supplements, drug therapies, or any other information from this book.

The author hereby specifically disclaims any and all liability arising directly or indirectly from the use or application of any of the products, ideas, procedures, drug therapies, or suggestions contained in this book and any errors, omissions, and inaccuracies in the information contained herein. The treatments and supplements included in this book are for identification purposes only and are not intended to recommend or endorse the product.

Preface

I discovered the importance of nutrition in 1978 at the age of twenty-two when my senior clinician at chiropractic school recommended I stop drinking milk and start taking betaine HCL with my meals. I was amazed and pleasantly surprised to find my digestive dysfunction and reoccurring urinary tract infections went away and never returned. One of my early mentors was Dr. M.T. Morter, Jr., who was president of Logan University while I attended and later authored several books. He was a proponent of alkalizing the body with foods and supplements that contained potassium, magnesium, zinc, selenium, and the like. One of the supplements I recommended in those days for my patients was *Green Magma*, a green powder made from barley sprouts, because of its mineral content. Generally speaking, the patient population of the late seventies and early eighties were a much healthier than the patients of today and needed less supplementation than the patients of today.

It has been known for some time that there have been significant mineral and vitamin deficiencies in the soil and the food sources in the United States for over eighty years. I found an interesting article from *Cosmopolitan* magazine concerning a report from Congress in 1936 about this mineral loss in the soil and foods in the U.S. (See this article in the Appendix.) Things have not gotten better since 1936, but have become worse, much worse. It is not a question if you have a nutritional deficiency—you do. It is more of a question of how many and how severe the deficiencies are.

Today, we have the technology to evaluate specific vitamin, mineral, amino acids, fatty acids, and anti-oxidants in individuals. There is no more guesswork in determining the specific nutritional needs of any individual.

This book builds on the data presented in Book 1, *13 Secrets of Optimal Aging.* If you have not yet read the first book in this series, I recommend that you do.

Table of Contents

Micronutrient Testing Introduction

Data in this book is organized by health problems, which are presented alphabetically. Micronutrient testing is a wonderful test—one I frequently recommend—and should be considered as a primary component of any preventative, wellness, or therapeutic treatment program. This test allows the clinician and patient to act as snipers in locating nutritional deficiencies instead of using a shotgun approach to nutritional supplementation.

The mineral content of our soil has been depleted by about 80% from the days of my great-grandparents and grandparents. The vitamin content of foods is dependent upon the mineral content in the food. Low mineral content in the soil equates to low mineral content in the fruits, vegetables, and grains and, therefore, low vitamin content as well. Even those individuals who eat only organic foods will have vitamin and mineral deficiencies. Because of what we have done to our soil, water, and air supply and the amount of toxic chemicals in the environment, nutraceutical supplementation is a must for optimum health. Even though nutrient levels are lower in our fruits and vegetables than they used to be, it is essential to eat these foods on a daily basis. Fresh fruits and vegetables are still far superior to any processed and packaged food. The sad truth is that even with our growing knowledge of the importance of good nutrition more Americans will go to bed tonight without having had a single serving of a fruit or vegetable.

One of the many challenges facing the clinician and the patient is determining what nutrients—vitamins, minerals, antioxidants, and fatty acids—that an individual needs. It is evident that we need to eat real, wholesome foods instead of packaged foods as much as possible. Generally speaking, most Americans eat too high a percentage of carbohydrates, particularly of the refined category. Certainly, as a general rule, most Americans do not eat enough vegetables. Most Americans are also lacking in good quality fatty acid intake coming from foods like avocadoes, nuts, seeds, olive oil, grass-fed beef, and ocean fish of the non-farm raised variety. Even with an optimum diet, which few of us have, nutritional deficiencies often occur due to the poor mineral content in the soil, which equates to lower vitamin, mineral, and antioxidant content in the foods, genetic variants that create a greater need for a particular nutrient, such as with the MTHFR (Methylenetetrahydrofolate reductase) gene variant and folate, and a high body burden of environmental toxins, such as mercury, lead, PCBs, PBAS, glyphosates (Roundup), and the like. Gene variants and environmental toxins create a greater need for specific micronutrients.

I want to re-emphasize the fact that the mineral content in the soil in North America is only about 1/7 of what it was just 100 years ago according to the World Health Organization in 2010. Accordingly, the micronutrient content of our foods is only 1/7 of what it was 100 years ago. Therefore, nutritional supplementation is a must as our requirements are way beyond what a synthetic one-a-day vitamin can provide. Most people have multiple nutrient deficiencies that are not met by this supplement. As much as possible, supplementation should come from whole food sources. There is a vast difference between ascorbic acid and a natural Vitamin C complex that also contains minerals and amino acids as well. There is also a difference between a natural vitamin and a synthetic vitamin. Naturally occurring vitamins are molecularly structured in what is known as a *cis* formation, while synthetic vitamins are in a *trans* formation. The body, in particular the cell membrane, is designed to recognize and accept the cis formation, not the trans. As a to be expected, the trans formation, synthetic vitamins are absorbed less efficiently, so you want to put methylated B vitamins in your body from food sources, not synthetic B vitamins made from coal tar.

Micronutrients—vitamins, minerals, amino acids, antioxidants, and fatty acids—are essential for proper enzyme function. Enzymes are bioelectric substances that transform one substance into another, taking away and/or adding molecules in the process. These enzymes are responsible for the transformation of one hormone into another as well as the breakdown and disposal of excess hormone in the blood. This process was discussed in *13 Secrets to Optimal Aging*, the first book in the *Health Restoration* series.

Micronutrients are also critical in supporting specific tissues. For example, all of the cells in the body need iodine, but the thyroid, breasts, uterus, and prostate require much more than other cells.

Embryologically speaking, the uterus in the woman and the prostate in the man come from the same tissue. When there is an iodine deficiency, these tissues suffer dysfunction, often noted by nodules, cysts, thickening, swelling, and the like. When there is a deficiency, the greater the need a tissue has for a particular nutrient the greater the amount of dysfunction. This is similar to the principle discussed in *13 Secrets to Optimal Aging.* The greater the number of receptor sites in a tissue or organ there are for a specific hormone the greater the need and dysfunction when there is a deficiency. As an example, the heart has more testosterone receptors in the body than anywhere else other than the testicles. Therefore, when testosterone drops dramatically, the heart is at increased risk for dysfunction and a heart attack.

Micronutrients additionally are essential to the mitochondrial energy chain The mitochondria of the cells is what turns the fatty acids from fats and the glucose from protein and carbohydrates in the food we eat into cellular energy. The making of this cellular energy is dependent upon multiple co-factors and numerous enzymatic transformations. Carnitine, an amino acid derivative, is a limiting factor in allowing fatty acids into the mitochondrial energy chain. Vitamins B1, B2, B3, B5, and lipoic acid are the limiting factors for allowing glucose into the mitochondrial energy chain. (See chart below.) Once the respective fuels, fatty acids or glucose, enter the mitochondria, there are multiple vitamins, minerals, and amino acids that are necessary to make the conversion into ATP (adenosine triphosphate). Some of these micronutrients are magnesium, manganese, iron, B6, B12, and coenzymeQ10.

Mitochondrial energy is essential for proper liver function to help detoxify the many chemicals in the air, water, and food and is necessary for ongoing cellular repair and maintenance. It is also required for clearing metabolic waste from the brain. Without adequate micronutrients, cell membranes, which consist of about 80% fat, cannot function properly. Adequate fatty acid intake is critical for optimal brain function. Cell membranes are responsible for taking in nutrients to make energy, maintenance and repair as well as disposing of cellular waste, taking in the good and getting rid of the bad. For example, glutamate, a primary stimulatory neurotransmitter, is dependent upon calcium, magnesium, and zinc to be adequate levels to be absorbed into the neuron. In essence, it

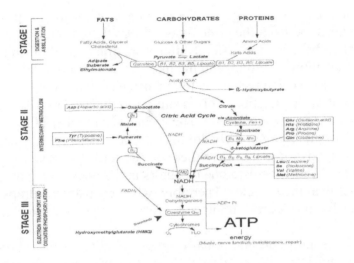

has a triple lock system: one for the calcium, one for the zinc, and one for the glutamate. This is discussed in more detail in the book *Saving Out Brains: Causes, Prevention, and Treatment for Dementia and Alzheimer's,* which will be released soon in the *Health Restoration* series.

There are other reasons nutritional deficiencies can occur in addition to inadequate intake of proper food. A functional deficiency can occur when a nutrient is present, but it may not be properly activated, not be appropriately localized into the cell, or not have sufficient cofactors to function at a normal level of activity. Underlying reasons for a functional nutritional deficiency include malabsorption from the gastrointestinal tract, lack of transportation to the appropriate tissue, inability to pass through the cell membrane, lack of intracellular activation storage, or a lack of concentration or activity of essential cofactors.

Eating a food or swallowing a pill does not ensure that cells can use those nutrients. The nutrient must pass through the stomach, be absorbed by the small intestine, pass through the liver, be taken by the blood to the cells in the body, and then must pass through the cell membrane, where other nutrients are needed as part of the recipe. To circumvent this process, I recommend sublingual and transdermal products that have liposome technology. Liposome technology encloses the nutrient or hormone with phosphatidylcholine, a naturally occurring fat found in the cell membrane. The cell membranes allow the liposome carrying the nutrient through more readily. Another good choice for taking nutraceuticals is isotonic preparations, which also allow for increased absorption.

By design, this used to be a somewhat simple process for an individual as long as s/he ate a variety of colorful and wholesome food. However, because of the amount of processed foods containing trans-fats, high fructose corn syrup, MSG, aspartame, and tens if not hundreds of other chemicals that the average person consumes on a daily basis, obtaining necessary nutrients is significantly more challenging these days. The more man-made chemicals we ingest the more nutrients we need to detoxify our bodies. This detoxification is in addition to the normal fuel a person needs every day for cellular energy to maintain, repair, and replicate his/her body.

Certain tissues contain and need more of a specific nutrient than other tissues. For example, every cell in the body needs iodine. However, the thyroid, breasts, uterus, and prostate contain the majority of this nutrient. When iodine levels are low, these tissues suffer greater dysfunction, causing symptoms that can manifest as nodules or goiter in the thyroid, lumps in the breast, uterine fibroids, or prostate enlargement. Both the uterus and prostate need a great amount of zinc compared to other tissues in the body. Deficiency of zinc can also cause similar symptoms in the prostate and uterus.

Key micronutrients are essential in the process of mitochondria energy production for ongoing cellular repair, maintenance, and duplication as well as the production of the many thousands of essential chemicals that cells make. For example, the parietal cell in the stomach is designed to make and secrete hydrochloric acid that then stimulates pancreatic enzymes and bile to be emptied into the small intestine, where absorption takes place. The parietal cells are dependent upon zinc and thiamine, a B Vitamin. Deficiencies of either can cause less hydrochloric acid to be secreted that, in turn, causes less pancreatic enzymes and bile to be secreted. The food is not well digested, and more deficiencies occur because the vitamins and minerals are not broken out from the protein in the food.

The beta cell in the pancreas produces insulin, which is necessary to transport the sugar (glucose) into the cells to be used for energy. The beta cell in the pancreas and the osteoblast, a new bone cell, are dependent upon Vitamin D (among many other nutrients) to function properly. If there is not adequate Vitamin D available, type

II diabetes or osteoporosis can manifest.

SpectraCell's micronutrient testing measures 33 specific nutrients, vitamins, minerals, amino acids, antioxidants, and metabolites that are essential contributors in mitochondrial energy production, the detoxification of dangerous hormone metabolites, the regulation of neurotransmitters, gene regulation, and hormone synthesis, and immune response.

This test includes assessment for **(vitamins)**—Vitamin A, Vitamins B1, B2, B3, B6, B12, biotin, folate, pantothenate, Vitamin C, Vitamin D, Vitamin K; **(minerals)**—calcium, magnesium, manganese, zinc, copper; **(amino acids)**—aspargine, glutamine, serine; **(fatty acids)**—oleic acid; **(antioxidants)**—alpha lipoic acid, coenzyme Q10, cysteine, glutathione, selenium, Vitamin E; **(metabolites)**—choline, inositol, carnitine; **(carbohydrate metabolism)**—chromium, fructose sensitivity, glucose-insulin metabolism; *Spectrox* (for total anti-oxidant function); and *Immudex* (immune response score).

Micronutrients Affect Many Functions in the Human Body

Micronutrients profoundly affect hormonal health. Conversely, hormones profoundly affect nutrient levels. The nutrient hormone interaction is quite intricate, so evaluating a one of the two in the context of the other provides a clearer picture of what is going on with each patient. The ways that micronutrients influence hormones are many and varied (See *13 Secrets to Optimal Aging—Book 1* of *Health Restoration* series.) Micronutrients act on hormone precursors. For example, Vitamin D, which is not a vitamin but actually a hormone, is also a hormone precursor for other steroid hormones.

Micronutrients also catalyze hormone synthesis. Zinc, for example, is a required co-factor in the synthesis of testosterone as well as over 300 other enzymatic functions. Similarly, selenium is required to convert thyroid hormone T4 into the biologically active hormone T3. The intermediary, androstenedione can either convert to testosterone or estrone. Decreased conversion to testosterone is related to deficiencies in Coenzyme Q10, alpha lipoic acid, Vitamin E, and zinc. Co-factor deficiencies directly impact hormone conversion and production.

The nutrient/hormone/enzyme relationship is both powerful and intricate. Micronutrients serve as strict components to hormones. Aspartic acid, an amino acid, is a key structural component of thyroid stimulating hormone (TSH). Micronutrients likewise regulate enzymes that act on hormones. As an example, Vitamin C inhibits aromatase, an enzyme that converts testosterone to estradiol. Vitamin C has also been shown to increase progesterone.

Micronutrients additionally detoxify dangerous hormone metabolites: Folic acid, B6, B12, as well as minerals like magnesium and antioxidants like glutathione, are needed to convert dangerous estrogen metabolites into benign or even beneficial metabolites. In fact, a deficiency of specific micronutrients increases the risk of certain cancers (breast, uterus, ovarian, prostate) through inefficient metabolism of carcinogenic estrogen by-products.

Micronutrients affect *neurotransmitters* that regulate hormones. A good example of this is the interaction of Vitamin B6, *prolactin*, and *dopamine*. Vitamin B6 is a co-factor for dopamine, which inhibits prolactin secretion, thus telling the pituitary to increase testosterone. Micronutrients—vitamins, minerals, and antioxidants--activate genes that regulate hormones and directly affect that genetic expression. For example, Vitamin A activates the gene that controls the release of thyroid-stimulating hormone.

Conversely, hormones alter nutrient levels and directly impact the function of several nutrients. For example, thyroid hormone stimulates the production of the copper transport protein, *ceruloplasmin*. Similarly, prolactin stimulates intestinal calcium absorption. The hormonal influence on micronutrients states is complex: Micronutrients are essential to the healthy tissue function of organs. The prostate gland has more zinc than any other tissues in the body. Zinc, involved in over 300 enzymatic reactions in the body, is essential in the production of HCL in the stomach and in immune response.

Micronutrients, in addition, are essential in the energy production within the mitochondria of the cells. Many of the B Vitamins, magnesium, Coenzyme Q10, and L-carnitine are all co-factors involved in this energy production. Deficiencies of any of these micronutrients inhibit energy production, contributing to cellular dysfunction of the liver and inhibiting detoxification processes. The lack of these co-factors also affects the ability of the heart to contract, reducing oxygenated blood throughout the body. SpectraCell's Micronutrients Testing provides the most comprehensive nutritional analysis available measuring functional deficiencies at the cellular level.

To make the relevance of nutritional deficiencies more real to you, let me show you what the research indicates concerning micronutrient deficiencies and some common conditions that you, your family, or friends might be suffering from.

ADHD

The diagnosis of Attention Deficit Disorder (ADHD) has increased since the middle of the last century. While the diagnosis is still controversial, there are numerous studies linking the symptoms of this disorder to nutritional deficiencies. Consequently, several vitamin deficiencies are associated with ADHD. Low folate status in pregnancy has been linked to hyperactivity in children. People with the MTHFR gene are predisposed to folate deficiency and, therefore, more likely to have ADHD.[1,2] Due to the role of Vitamin B6 in raising serotonin levels, supplementation of high doses of Vitamin B6 has been shown to be as effective as Ritalin for ADHD, or at least that is what the evidence supports.[3,4,5] The B Vitamin choline is the precursor to the neurotransmitter acetylcholine, which regulates memory, focus, and muscle control related to hyperactivity. [6,7]

There are also several mineral deficiencies related to this condition. For example, a magnesium deficiency is linked to poor function of the neurotransmitters that control emotion, social reactions, hyperactivity, and attention. This mineral exhibits a synergistic effect with Vitamin B6.[8,9,10] Zinc is a cofactor for dopamine synthesis that affects mood and concentration in ADHD. Low zinc depresses both melatonin and serotonin production, which affect information processing and behavior in ADHD.[11,12,13,14]

Carnitine, an amino acid, reduces hyperactivity and improves social behavior in people with ADHD due to its role in fatty acid metabolism. This is a possible safe alternative to stimulant drugs, and it has none of the side effects of stimulants.[15,16,17] Often, nutrients work better in the presence of other nutrients. The administration of phosphatidylserine, a source of serine, with omega 3 fatty acids improved the attention scores of people with ADHD significantly better than omega 3 fatty acids alone. Phosphatidylserine increases dopamine levels, which improve emotional levels.[18, 19-21] It also is the glutamine precursor for the calming neurotransmitter GABA (gamma-aminobutyric acid) that affects mood, focus, and hyperactivity. Disruption of the glutamine-containing neurotransmission systems may be a cause of ADHD,[22-24] and a deficiency of glutathione is common in this condition.[24,25] Also, oxidative imbalance is prevalent in ADHD patients and likely plays a causative role.[26,27]

Reference List

1. Krull R, Brouwers P, Jain N, et al. Folate pathway genetic polymorphisms are related to attention disorders in childhood leukemia survivors. *J Pediatr* 2008;152:101-105.
2. Schlotz W, Jones A, Phillips D, et al. Lower maternal folate status in early pregnancy is associated with childhood hyperactivity and peer problems in offspring. *J Child Psychol Psychiatry* 2010;51:594-602.
3. Coleman M, Steinberg J, Tippett J, et al. A preliminary study of the effect of pyridoxine administration in a subgroup of hyperkinetic children: a double-blind crossover comparison with methylphenidate. *Biol Psychiatry* 1979;14:741-751.
4. Mousain-Bosc M, Roche M, Polge A, et al. Improvement of neurobehavioral disorders in children supplemented with magnesium-vitamin B6. I. Attention deficit hyperactivity disorders. *Magnes Res* 2006;19:46-52.
5. Mousain-Bosc M, Roche M, Rapin J, et al. Magnesium and Vitamin B6 intake reduces central nervous system hyperexcitability in children. *J Am Coll Nutr* 2004;23:545S-548S.
6. Barth V, Need A, Tzavara E, et al. In vivo occupancy of dopamine D3 receptors by antagonists produces neurochemical and behavioral effects of potential relevance to attention-deficit-hyperactivity disorder. *J Pharmacol Exp Ther* 2013; 344:501-510
7. English B, Hahn M, Gizer I, et al. Choline transporter gene variation is associated with attention-deficit hyperactivity disorder. *J Neurodev Disord* 2009;1:252-263.
8. Huss M, Volp A, Stauss-Grabo M. Supplementation of polyunsaturated fatty acids, magnesium and zinc in children seeking medical advice for attention-deficit/hyperactivity problems - an observational cohort study. *Lipids Health Dis* 2010;9:105.
9. Arnold L, DiSilvestro R. Zinc in attention-deficit/hyperactivity disorder. *J Child Adolesc Psychopharmacol* 2005;15:619-627.
10. Yorbik O, Ozdag M, Olgun A, et al. Potential effects of zinc on information processing in boys with attention deficit

hyperactivity disorder. *Prog Neuropsychopharmacol Biol Psychiatry* 2008;32:662- 667.

11. Arnold L, Pinkham S, Votolato N. Does zinc moderate essential fatty acid and amphetamine treatment of attention-deficit/hyperactivity disorder? *J Child Adolesc Pychopharmacol* 2000;10:111-117.

12. Dodig-Curkovic K, Dovhanj J, Curkovic M, et al. The role of zinc in the treatment of hyperactivity disorder in children. *Acta Med Croatica* 2009;63:307-313.

13. Arnold L, Amato A, Bozzolo H, et al. Acetyl-L-carnitine (ALC) in attention-deficit/hyperactivity disorder: a multi-site, placebo-controlled pilot trial. *J Child Adolesc Psychopharmacol* 2007;17:791-802.

14. Van Oudheusden L. Scholte H. Efficacy of carnitine in the treatment o children with attention-deficit hyperactivity disorder. *Prostaglandins Leukot Essent Fatty Acids* 2002;67:33-38.

15. Torrioli M, Vernacotola S, Peruzzi L, et al. A double blind, parallel, multicenter comparison of L-acetylcarnitine with placebo on the attention deficit hyperactivity disorder in fragile X syndrome boys. *Am J Med Genet* 2008;146:803.812.

16. Kidd P. Omega-3 DHA and EPA for cognition, behavior, and mood: clinical findings and structural-functional synergies with cell membrane phospholipids. *Altern Med Rev* 2007;12:207-227.

17. Vaisman N, Kaysar N, Zaruk-Adasha Y, et al. Correlation between changes in blood fatty acid composition and visual sustained attention performance in children with inattention: effect of dietary n-3 fatty acids containing phospholipids. *Am J Clin Nutr* 2008;87:1170-1180.

18. SpectraCell Laboratories. *ADHD.* http://www.healthbean.ca/wp-content/uploads/2015/03/ADHD.pdf. 2013. Accessed 20 Sep 2016.

19. Pellow J, Solomon E, Barnard C. Complementary and alternative medical therapies for children with attention-deficit/hyperactivity disorder (ADHD). *Altern Med Rev* 2011;16:323-337.

---

20. Perlov E, Philipsen A, Hesslinger B, et al. Reduced cingulated glutamate/glutamine-to-creatine ratios in adult patients with attention deficit/hyperactivity disorder – a magnetic resonance spectroscopy study. *J Psychiatr Res* 2007;41:934-941.
21. Carrey N, MacMaster F, Gaudet L, et al. Striatal creatine and glutamate/glutamine in attentiondeficit/hyperactivity disorder. *J Child Adolesc Psychopharmacol* 2007; 17:11-17.
22. Rusch N, Boeker M, Buchert M, et al. Neurochemical alterations in women with borderline personality disorder and comorbid attention-deficit hyperactivity disorder. *World J Biol Psychiatry* 2010;11: 372-381.
23. Kronenberg G, Ende G, Alm B, et al. Increased NAA and reduced choline levels in the anterior cingulum following chronic methylphenidate. A spectroscopic test-retest study in adult ADHD. *Eur Arch Psychiatry Clin Neurosci* 2008;258:446-450.
24. Dvorakova M, Sivonova M, Trebaticka J, et al. The effect of polyphenolic extract from pine bark, Pycnogenol on the level of glutathione in children suffering from attention deficit hyperactivity disorder (ADHD). *Redox Rep* 2008;11:163-172.
25. Bulut M, Selek S, Gergerlioglu H, et al. Malondialdehyde levels in adult attention-deficit hyperactivity disorder. *J Psychiatry Neurosci* 2007;32:435-438.
26. Selek S. Savas H, Gergerlioglu H, et al. Oxidative imbalance in adult attention deficit/hyperactivity disorder. *Biol Psychol* 2008;79:256-259.
27. Spahis S, Vanasse M, Belanger S, et al. Lipid profile, fatty acid composition and pro- and anti-oxidant status in pediatric patients with attention-deficit/hyperactivity disorder. *Prostaglandins Leukot Essent Fatty Acids* 2008;79:47-53.

Additional references at **http://www.spectracell.com/online-library-mnt-adhd-abstracts/**
(Some content Adapted from SpectraCell Laboratories, Inc.)

Anxiety

Anxiety is defined as a feeling of worry, nervousness, or unease, typically about an imminent event or something with an uncertain outcome. Nutritional deficiencies may be linked to these feelings. There is one important B Vitamin that affects feelings of anxiety. Inositol is a neurochemical messenger in the brain, and it (Vitamin B8) affects dopamine and serotonin receptors. Clinical trials confirm taking this supplement is very effective in reducing panic attacks.[1,2] Another B, choline, is a precursor to the neurotransmitter acetylcholine, which affects focus and mood. Low levels of choline have been linked to anxiety.[3,4]

Vitamin B6 is a cofactor in synthesis of calming neurotransmitters, such as GABA (gamma-aminobutyric acid), serotonin and dopamine.[5-7] Anxiety is a symptom of severe B3 (niacin) deficiency, which also can cause pellagra. Vitamin B3 is another cofactor for the synthesis of calming neurotransmitters. When taken in doses sufficient to create a therapeutic effect, it may enhance the calming effects of GABA in the brain. B3 also converts tryptophan to serotonin.[8,9] Another B Vitamin, folate, aids in production of neurotransmitters, such as dopamine and serotonin, which have a calming effect on mood.[10,11] Additionally, low Vitamin D status is linked to anxiety.[12,13] Animal studies confirm the role of Vitamins D and E in reducing anxiety-related behavior.[14, 15]

The mineral copper is an integral part of certain chemicals in the brain, such as endorphins, that calm anxious feelings. Anxiety-like behavior may be exacerbated with copper deficiency.[16-18] Another mineral, magnesium, regulates the HPA (hypothalamic-pituitary-adrenal) axis, which controls physical and psychological reactions to stress. A magnesium deficiency can induce anxiety and emotional hyper-reactivity.[19-21] Selenium repletion to normal levels reduced anxiety scores in clinical trials. Some studies suggest the mechanism of action is due to its role in key regulatory proteins called selenoproteins.[22-23] Zinc has reduced anxiety in clinical trials, possibly due to its interaction with NMDA (N-methyl-D- aspartate) receptors in the brain, which regulate mood.[24,25] Chromium's effect on serotonin transmission may explain its anxiolytic (anxiety relieving) effect in animal studies.[26,27]

Finally, studies show that carnitine, an amino acid, can reduce anxiety and improve feelings of well-being.[28,29] Serine, another amino acid, exerts a calming effect by buffering the adrenal response to physical or emotional stress. It has been shown to lower anxiety scores of patients with post-traumatic stress disorder.[30-32]

Reference List

1. Bejamin J, Levine J, Fux M, et al. Double-blind, placebo-controlled, crossover trial of inositol treatment for panic disorder. *Am J Psychiatry* 1995;152:1084-1086.
2. Palatnik A, Frolov K, Fux M et al. Double-blind, controlled, crossover trial of inositol versus fluvoxamine for the treatment of panic disorder. *J Clin Psychopharmacol* 2001;21:335-339.
3. Bjelland I, Tell G, Vollset S, et al. Choline in anxiety and depression: the Hordaland Health Study. *Am J Clin Nutr* 2009;90:1056-1060.
4. Martinowich K, Schloesser RJ, Lu Y, et al. Roles of p75(NTR), long-term depression, and cholinergic transmission in anxiety and acute stress coping. *Biol Pyschiatry* 2012;71:75-83.
5. Head K, Kelly G. Nutrients and botanicals for treatment of stress: adrenal fatigue, neurotransmitter imbalance, anxiety, and restless sleep. *Altern Med Rev* 2009;14:114-140.
6. McCarty M. High-does pyridoxine as an 'anti-stress' strategy. *Med Hypotheses* 2000;54:803-807.
7. Baldewicz T, Goodkin K, Feaster DJ, et al. Plasma pyridoxine deficiency is related to increased psychological distress in recently bereaved homosexual men. *Psychosom Med* 1998;60:297-308.
8. Prousky J. Niacinamide's potent role in alleviating anxiety with its benzodiazepine-like properties: a case report. *J Orthomolec Med* 2004;19:104-110.
9. Prakash R, Gandotra S, Singh L, et al. Rapid resolution of delusional parasitosis in pellagra with niacin augmentation therapy. *Gen Hosp Psychiatry* 2008;30:581-584.
10. Kelly G. Folates: Supplemental Forms and Therapeutic Applications. *Altern Med Rev*1998;3:208-220.
11. Ferguson S, Berry K, Hansen D, et al. Behavioral effects of prenatal folate deficiency in mice. *Birth Defects Res A Clin Mol Teratol* 2005;73:249-252.

12. Kalueff A, Lou R, Lasski I, et al. Increased anxiety in mice lacking vitamin D receptor gene. *Neuroreport* 2004;15:1271-1274.
13. Armstrong D, Meenagh G, Bickle I, et al. Vitamin D deficiency is associated with anxiety and depression in fibromyalgia. *Clin Rheumatol* 2007;26:551-554.
14. Terada Y, Okura Y, Kikusui T, et al. Dietary vitamin E deficiency increases anxiety-like behavior in juvenile and adult rats. *Biosci Biotechnol Biochem* 2011;75:1894-1899.
15. Okura Y, Tawara S, Kikusui T, et al. Dietary vitamin E deficiency increases anxiety-related behavior in rats under stress of social isolation. *Biofactors* 2009;35:273-278.
16. Bargellini A, Piccinini L, De Palma M, et al. Trace elements, anxiety and immune parameters in patients affected by cancer. *J Trace Elem Med Biol* 2003;17 Suppl 1:3-9.
17. Bousquet-Moore D, Prohaska J, Nillni E, et al. Interactions of peptide amidation and copper: novel biomarkers and mechanisms of neural dysfunction. *Neurobiol Dis* 2010;37:130-140.
18. Railey A, Micheli T, Wanschura P, et al. Alterations in fear response and spatial memory in pre and post-natal zinc supplemented rats: remediation by copper. *Physiol Behav* 2010;100:95-100.
19. Sartori SB, Whittle N, Hetzenauer A, et al. Magnesium deficiency induces anxiety and HPA axis dysregulation: modulation by therapeutic drug treatment. *Neuropharmacology* 2012;62:304-312.
20. Fromm L, Heath D, Vink R, et al. Magesium attenuates post-traumatic depression/ anxiety following diffuse traumatic brain injury in rats. *J Am Coll Nutr* 2004;23:529S-533S.
21. Poleszak E, Szewczyk B, Kedzierska E, et al. Antidepressant- and anxiolytic-like activity of magnesium in mice. *Pharmacol Biochem Behav* 2004;78:7-12.
22. Shor-Posner G, Lecusay R, Miguez MJ, et al. Psychological burden in the era of HAART: impact of selenium therapy. *Int J Psychiatry Med* 2003;33:55-69.
23. Benton D, Cook R. The impact of selenium supplementation on mood. *Biol Psychiatry* 1991;29:1092-1098.

24. Joshi M, Akhtar M, Najmi A, et al. Effect of zinc in animal models of anxiety, depression and psychosis. *Hum Exp Toxicol* 2012;Epub ahead of print.
25. Cope E, Levenson C. Role of zinc in the development and treatment of mood disorders. *Curr Opin Clin Nutr Metab Care* 2010;13:685-689.
26. Partyka A, Jastrzębska-Więsek M, Szewczyk B, et al. Anioxyltic-like activity of zinc in rodent tests. *Pharmacol Re.* 2011;63:1050-5.
27. Khanam R, Pillai K. Effect of chronic chromium picolinate in animal models of anxiety and memory. *Fundam Clin Pharmacol* 2007;21:531-534.
28. Khanam R, Pillai K. Effect of chromium picolinate on modified forced swimming test in diabetic rats: involvement of serotonergic pathways and potassium channels. *Basic Clin Pharmacol Toxicol* 2006;98:155-159.
29. Levine J, Kaplan Z, Pettegrew J, et al. Effect of intraperitoneal acetyl-L-carnitine (ALCAR) on anxiety-like behaviours in rats. *Int J Neuropsychopharmacol* 2005;8:65-74.
30. Malaguarnera M, Bella R, Vacante M, et al. Acetyl-L-carnitine reduces depression and improves quality of life in patients with minimal hepatic encephalopathy. *Scand J Gastroenterology* 2011;46:750-759.
31. Heresco-Levy U, Vass A, Bloch B, et al. Pilot controlled trial of d-serine for the treatment of posttraumatic stress disorder. *Int J Neuropsychopharmacol* 2009;12:1279-1282.
32. de Koning T, Klomp L. Serine-deficiency syndromes. *Curr Opin Neurol* 2004;17:197-204.
33. Hellhammer J, Fries E, Buss C, et al. Effects of soy lecithin phosphatidic acid and phosphatidylserine complex (PAS) on the endocrine and psychological responses to mental stress. *Stress* 2004;7:119-126.

Additional references at **http://www.spectracell.com/online-library-mnt-anxiety-abstract/**
(Some content Adapted from SpectraCell Laboratories, Inc.)

Asthma

Asthma is a respiratory condition marked by spasms in the bronchi of the lungs that cause difficulty in breathing. These attacks are often triggered by allergens or environmental elements. The incidence of asthma is increasing in the U.S., particularly among those from low-income backgrounds.[1] There are several vitamins, minerals, and amino acids that influence this condition.

Studies indicate that deficiencies in some B vitamins relate to an asthmatic condition. Low folate status is linked to severity of an allergic response. In general, folate plays a key role in cellular immunity.[2,3] Additionally, animal and human studies show that taking choline strongly suppresses oxidative stress in lung tissue caused by asthma.[4,5] Vitamin B6 binds with the chemical (histamine) that causes airway constriction and inactivates it. Regrettably, the common asthma drug theophylline depletes B6.[6,7]

Vitamins E fights inflammatory enzymes in pulmonary epithelial tissue (inside surface of lungs) that cause asthmatic symptoms.[8-11] Higher levels of Vitamin D increases lung capacity in asthmatics while a deficiency increases severity of asthma attacks.[12-14] Vitamin C dilates bronchial airways and inhibits histamine-induced constriction of airways. It is needed for production of epinephrine, which mitigates asthma attacks.[15,16] Finally, Vitamin A prevents exercise-induced asthma and regulates bronchial responsiveness.[17,18]

As with several other conditions, magnesium, selenium, and zinc are important to preventing attacks. Magnesium promotes relaxation of bronchial smooth muscle and inhibits histamine release. It also reduces the tendency to develop anaphylaxis. Low intracellular levels of magnesium have been linked to asthma severity.[19-22] Selenium is part of the enzyme called glutathione peroxidase that protects against asthmatic lung tissue damage. Supplementation trials have been promising.[23-26] Since zinc regulates the immune system, including allergic response, a deficiency can exacerbate asthma symptoms.[27,28]

Deficiencies in amino acids may engender asthmatic symptoms. Carnitine protects the surface of the lungs while it improves pulmonary function in asthmatics by decreasing inflammation in lung tissue.[29-31] The antioxidant Coenzyme Q10 (CoQ10) needs to be replenished if there have been steroid medications prescribed for asthma because they cause damage to the mitochondria, the site of cellular energy production. CoQ10 repairs this damage and may reduce corticosteroid dosage in asthmatics.[32,33]

Reference List

1. United States Environmental Protection Agency. *Asthma Facts.* https://www.epa.gov/sites/production/files/2015-10/documents/asthma_fact_sheet_eng_july_30_2015_v2.pdf. Aug 2015. Accessed 21 Sep 2016.
2. Matsui E, Matsui W. Higher serum folate levels are associated with a lower risk of atopy and wheeze. *J Allergy Clin Immunol* 2009;123:1253-1259.
3. Farres M, Shahin R, Melek N, et al. Study of folate status among Egyptian asthmatics. *Intern Med* 2011;50:205-211.
4. Mehta A, Arora N, Gaur S, et al. Choline supplementation reduces oxidative stress in mouse model of allergic airway disease. *Eur J Clin Invest* 2009;39:934-941.
5. Mehta A, Singh B, Arora N, et al. Choline attenuates immune inflammation and suppresses oxidative stress in patients with asthma. *Immunobiology* 2010;215:527-534.
6. Wu F, Christen P, Gehring H. A novel approach to inhibit intracellular vitamin B6-dependent enzymes: proof of principle with human and plasmodium ornithine decarboxylase and human histidine decarboxylase. *FASEB J* 2011;25:109-122.
7. Shimizu T, Maeda S, Mochizuki H, et al. Theophylline attenuates circulating vitamin B6 levels in children with asthma. *Pharmacology* 1994;49:392-397.
8. Wang Y, Moreland M, Wagner J, et al. Vitamin E forms inhibit IL-13/STAT6-induced eotaxin-3 secretion by up-regulation of PAR4, an endogenous inhibitor of atypical PKC in human lung epithelial cells. *J Nutr Biochem* 2012;23:602-608.
9. Hoskins A, Roberts J, Milne G, et al. Natural-source d-α-tocopheryl acetate inhibits oxidant stress and modulates atopic asthma in humans in vivo. *Allergy* 2012;67:676-682.
10. Centanni S, Santus P, Di Marco F, et al. The potential role of tocopherol in asthma and allergies: modification of the leukotriene pathway. *BioDrugs* 2001;15:81-86.
11. Lim y, Vasu V, Valacchi G, et al. Severe vitamin E

deficiency modulates airway allergic inflammatory responses in the murine asthma model. *Free Radic Res* 2008;42:387-396.

12. Chinelllato I, Piazza M, Sandri M, et al. Vitamin D serum levels and markers of asthma control in Italian children. *J Pediatr* 2011;158:437-441.

13. Brehm J, Schuemann B, Fuhlbrigge A, et al. Serum vitamin D levels and severe asthma exacerbations in the Childhood Asthma Management Program study. *J Allergy Clin Immunol* 2010;126:52-58.

14. Wu A, Tantisira K, Li L, et al. The effect of vitamin D and inhaled corticosteroid treatment on lung function in children. *Am J Respir Crit Care Med* 2012; epub ahead of print.

15. Tecklenburg S, Mickleborough T, Fly A, et al. Ascorbic acid supplementation attenuates exercise-induced bronchoconstriction in patients with asthma. *Respir Med* 2007;101:1770-1778.

16. Ness A, Khaw K, et al. Vitamin C status and respiratory function. *Eur J Clin Nutr* 1996;50:573-579.

17. Neuman I, Nahum H, Ben-Amotz A. Prevention of exercise-induced asthma by a natural isomer mixture of beta-carotene. *Ann Allergy Asthma Immunol* 1999;82:549-553.

18. McGowan S, Smith J, Holmes A, et al. Vitamin A deficiency promotes bronchial hyperreactivity in rats by altering muscarinic M(2) receptor function. *Am J Physiol Lung Cell Mol Physiol* 2002;282:L1031-1039.

19. Kazaks A, Uriu-Adams J, Albertson T, et al. Effect of oral magnesium supplementation on measures of airway resistance and subjective assessment of asthma control and quality of life in men and women with mild to moderate asthma: a randomized placebo controlled trial. *J Asthma* 2010;47:83-92.

20. Ashkenazy Y, Moshonov S, Fischer G, et al. Magnesium-deficient diet aggravates anaphylactic shock and promotes cardiac myolysis in guinea pigs. *Magnes Trace Elem* 1990;9:283-288.

21. Alamoudi O. Hypomagnesaemia in chronic, stable asthmatics: prevalence, correlation with severity and hospitalization. *Eur Respir J* 2000;16:427-431.

22. Emelyanov A, Fedoseev G, Barnes P. Reduced intracellular

magnesium concentrations in asthmatic patients. *Eur Respir J* 1999;13:38-40.

23. Gazdik F, Kadrabova J, Gasdikova K. Decreased consumption of corticosteroids after selenium supplementation in corticoid-dependent asthmatics. *Bratisl Lek Listy* 2002;103:22-25.

24. Hasselmark L, Malmgren R, Zetterstrom O, et al. Selenium supplementation in intrinsic asthma. *Allergy*1993;48:30-36.

25. Norton R, Hoffmann P. Selenium and asthma. *Mol Aspects Med* 2012;33:98-106

26. Hoffmann P, Jourdan-Le Saux C, Hoffmann F, et al. A role for dietary selenium and selenoproteins in allergic airway inflammation. *J Immunol* 2007;179:3258-3267.

27. Morgan C, Ledford J, Zhou P, et al. Zinc supplementation alters airway inflammation and airway hyperresponsiveness to a common allergen. *J Inflamm* 2011;8:36

28. Murgia C, Grosser D, Truong-Tran A, et al. Apical localization of zinc transporter ZnT4 in human airway epithelial cells and its loss in a murine model of allergic airway inflammation. *Nutrients* 2011;3:910-928.

29. Al-Biltagi M, Isa M, Bediwy A, et al. L-carnitine improves the asthma control in children with moderate persistent asthma. *J Allergy* 2012;509730.

30. Asilsov S, Bekem O, Karaman O, et al. Serum total and free carnitine levels in children with asthma. *World J Pediatr* 2009;5:60-62.

31. Uzuner N, Kavukcu S, Yilmaz O, et al. The role of L-carnitine in treatment of a murine model of asthma. *Acta Med Okayama* 2002;56:295-301.

32. Gvozdjakova A, Kucharska J, Bartkovjakova M, et al. Coenzyme Q10 supplementation reduces corticosteroids dosage in patients with bronchial asthma. *Biofactors* 2005;25:235-240.

33. Gazdik F, Gvozdjakova A, Nadvornikova R, et al. Decreased levels of coenzyme Q(10) in patients with bronchial asthma. *Allergy* 2002;57:811-814.

Additional references at **http://www.spectracell.com/online-library-mnt-asthma-abstract**
(Some content Adapted from SpectraCell Laboratories, Inc.)

Autism

There has been an unprecedented rise in autism in recent years. Although many factors likely have contributed to the rise in numbers for autism, compelling evidence suggests that nutritional deficiencies along with multiple environmental toxins may be a contributing factor.

Supplementation with Vitamin B1 (thiamine) has shown a positive effect for some autistic children in the area of language acquisition.[1,2] A deficiency in Vitamin B1 has been associated with delayed language development in childhood. Since the brain is quite vulnerable to biotin (Vitamin B7) deficiency, a deficiency can potentially cause neurological problems associated with autism.[3] Low levels of Vitamin D have also been linked with autism.[4,5] In some cases of severe deficiency, high-dose Vitamin D therapy reversed some of the autistic behaviors.[6]

As with many nutrients, magnesium and Vitamin B6 work together to improve clinical symptoms of autism.[7] When one group of autistic children was supplemented with magnesium and Vitamin B6, 70% of the children showed improvement in social interaction and communication.[8] As might be predicted, when the supplements were stopped, the clinical symptoms reappeared. In another study, physical aggression and inattention improved after supplementation with magnesium and Vitamin B6 for a few months.[9] Another important mineral related to autism is zinc since zinc levels are much lower in autistic individuals.[10,11] Zinc is indispensable for proper elimination of the toxic metal mercury from brain tissue, a condition that has also been linked to autism.[12]

The brain and nerves are composed mostly of fat. The most important of these fats are called omega-3 fatty acids, found primarily in fish or fish oil supplements. These are so essential that they must be present throughout a lifetime. Also called EPA and DHA, they are absolutely essential for human health, and their concentration in the brain makes them superstars in neurological disorders, such as autism. Mounting evidence implicates deficiencies in omega-3 fatty acids for the rise in autism.[13,14]

Deficiencies in amino acids contribute to autism. For example, levels of the amino acids glutamine and asparagine are lower in autistic children.[15,16] Autistic individuals have significantly reduced carnitine, another amino acid, whose primary function is to transport fatty acids like omega-3 fatty acids into cells so they can be used for energy. This reduction then affects the patient's ability to use the fatty acids that are so critical to his/her learning and social development.[17]

Oxidative stress is a term used to describe damage to cells that occurs on a daily basis throughout the body. Fortunately, bodies have built-in defenses against the onslaught of internal and external toxins causing oxidative stress in tissues. Not too surprising, several studies show an increase in oxidative stress in autism, resulting in an impaired ability to eliminate toxins. One study associated damage in fatty tissue surrounding cells to symptoms of autism.[18-20]

Reference List

1. Obrenovich ME, Shola D, Schroedel K, Agrahari A, Lonsdale D. The role of trace elements, thiamin (e) and transketolasen autism and autistic spectrum disorder. *Front Biosci* (Elite Ed). 2015 Jan 1;7:229-41. Review. PMID: 25553376

2. Lonsdale D, Shamberger RJ, Audhya T. Treatment of autism spectrum children with thiamine tetrahydrofurfuryl disulfide: a pilot study. *Neuro Endocrinol Lett*. 2002 Aug;23(4):303-8. PMID: 12195231.

3. Zaffanello M[1], Zamboni G, Fontana E, Zoccante L, Tatò L. A case of partial biotinidase deficiency associated with autism.*Child Neuropsychol*. 2003 Sep;9(3):184-8.

4. Shan L, Hu XL, Wang B, Jia FY. Research advances in the role of vitamin D in autism spectrum disorders. *Zhongguo Dang Dai Er Ke Za Zhi*. 2016 Feb;18(2):183-8. *Review*. Chinese. PMID: 26903068.

5. Stubbs G, Henley K, Green J. Autism: Will vitamin D supplementation during pregnancy and early childhood reduce the recurrence rate of autism in newborn siblings? *J. Med Hypotheses*. 2016 Mar;88:74-8. doi: 10.1016/j.mehy.2016.01.015. Epub 2016 Feb 2. PMID: 26880644

6. Feng J, Shan L, Du L, Wang B, Li H, Wang W, Wang T, Dong H, Yue X, Xu Z, Staal WG, Jia F Clinical improvement following vitamin D3 supplementation

in Autism Spectrum Disorder. *Nutr Neurosci.* 2016 Jan 18. [Epub ahead of print]. PMID: 26783092.

7. Murza KA, Pavelko SL, Malani MD, Nye C. Vitamin B6-magnesium treatment for autism: the current status of the research. *Magnes Res.* 2010 Jun;23(2):115-7. doi: 10.1684/mrh.2010.0209. Epub 2010 Jun 18. Review. No abstract available. PMID: 20562088.

8. Mousain-Bosc M, Roche M, Polge A, Pradal-Prat D, Rapin J, Bali JP. Improvement of neurobehavioral disorders in children supplemented with magnesium-vitamin B6. II. Pervasive developmental disorder-autism. *Magnes Res.* 2006 Mar;19(1):53-62. PMID: 16846101.

9. Nye C, Brice A. Combined vitamin B6-magnesium treatment in autism spectrum disorder. *Cochrane Database Syst Rev.* 2005 Oct 19;(4):CD003497. Review. PMID: 16235322.

10. Crăciun EC, Bjørklund G, Tinkov AA, Urbina MA, Skalny AV, Rad F, Dronca E. Evaluation of whole blood zinc and copper levels in children with autism spectrum disorder. *Metab Brain Dis.* 2016 Aug;31(4):887-90. doi: 10.1007/s11011-016-9823-0. Epub 2016 Apr 8. PMID: 27059237.

11. The role of zinc and copper in autism spectrum disorders. *Bjorklund G.Acta Neurobiol Exp* (Wars). 2013;73(2):225-36. Review. PMID: 23823984.

12. Kern JK, Geier DA, Sykes LK, Haley BE, Geier MR. The relationship between mercury and autism: A comprehensive review and discussion. *J Trace Elem Med Biol.* 2016 Sep;37:8-24. doi: 10.1016/j.jtemb.2016.06.002. Epub 2016 Jun 2. Review. PMID: 27473827.

13. van Elst K, Bruining H, Birtoli B, Terreaux C, Buitelaar JK, Kas MJ.Food for thought: dietary changes in essential fatty acid ratios and the increase in autism spectrum disorders. *Neurosci Biobehav Rev.* 2014 Sep;45:369-78. doi:10.1016/j.neubiorev.2014.07.004. Epub 2014 Jul 12. Review. PMID: 25025657.

14. Autism as a disorder of deficiency of brain-derived neurotrophic factor and altered metabolism of polyunsaturated fatty acids. *Das UN Nutrition.* 2013 Oct;29(10):1175-85. doi: 10.1016/j.nut.2013.01.012. Epub 2013 Jul 30. Review. PMID:23911220.

---

15. Cochran DM, Sikoglu EM, Hodge SM, Edden RA, Foley A, Kennedy DN, Moore CM, Frazier JA. Relationship among Glutamine, γ-Aminobutyric Acid, and Social Cognition in Autism Spectrum Disorders. *J Child Adolesc Psychopharmacol.* 2015 May;25(4):314-22. doi: 10.1089/cap.2014.0112. Epub 2015 Apr 28. PMID: 25919578.
16. Naushad SM, Jain JM, Prasad CK, Naik U, Akella RR. Autistic children exhibit distinct plasma amino acid profile. *Indian J Biochem Biophys.* 2013 Oct;50(5):474-8. PMID: 24772971.
17. Mostafa GA, Al-Ayadhi LY. Reduced levels of plasma polyunsaturated fatty acids and serum carnitine in autistic children: relation to gastrointestinal manifestations. *Behav Brain Funct.* 2015 Feb 7;11:4. doi: 10.1186/s12993-014-0048-2. PMID: 25757041.
18. Cortelazzo A, De Felice C, Guerranti R, et al. Expression and oxidative modifications of plasma proteins in autism spectrum disorders: Interplay between inflammatory response and lipid peroxidation. *Proteomics Clin Appl.* 2016 Jun 1. doi: 10.1002/prca.201500076. [Epub ahead of print] PMID: 27246309
19. Yui K, Kawasaki Y, Yamada H, Ogawa S. Oxidative Stress and Nitric Oxide in Autism Spectrum Disorder and Other Neuropsychiatric Disorders. *CNS Neurol Disord Drug Targets.* 2016;15(5):587-96.PMID:27071787.
20. Menezo YJ, Elder K, Dale B. Link Between Increased Prevalence of Autism Spectrum Disorder Syndromes and Oxidative Stress, DNA Methylation, and Imprinting: The Impact of the Environment. *JAMA Pediatr.* 2015 Nov;169(11):1066-7. doi: 10.1001/jamapediatrics.2015.2125. No abstract available. PMID: 26414354.

(Some content Adapted from SpectraCell Laboratories, Inc.)

Breast Health

Every woman is biochemically unique, and several factors—age, lifestyle, metabolism, prescription drug usage, past and present illnesses, absorption rate, genetics and more—affect her personal nutritional needs. Prevention is more than earlier diagnosis. True prevention starts with your body's foundation—micronutrients. Research shows that micronutrients assist in repairing cellular damage in breast tissue, the prevention of genetic mutations, and maintaining healthy hormonal balance.

Several vital nutrients are critical for maintaining healthy breast tissue. Vitamin A mitigates DNA damage in cancerous tissue and inhibits hormonal toxicities that can initiate cancerous cells.[1,2] Vitamin D enhances breast health by lowering the risk of breast cancer by 70%.[3] B Vitamins, especially folic acid, may prevent mutations in breast tissue that eventually become carcinogenic.[4] Deficiencies of specific B Vitamins—folate, B6, and B 12—and the amino acid glutathione contribute to formation of bad estrogens, a known carcinogen.[6,7]

Unfortunately, research indicates that synthetic hormone replacement therapy affects minerals, such as calcium, copper, chromium, magnesium, selenium and zinc.[8] Calcium works with Vitamin D to enhance breast health.[9] Low antioxidant status is connected to higher rates of breast and other cancers.[10,11] In reality, antioxidants, such as coenzyme Q10, cysteine, and previously mentioned Vitamin A, have been shown to reduce DNA damage in cancerous tissue and prevent the toxicity of estrogen that often causes cancerous cells.[12,13]

Minerals, vitamins, antioxidants, and metabolites interact closely with hormones. Improving estrogen metabolism, which is highly dependent on the availability of specific nutrients, reduces the risk of many hormone related cancers, including breast cancer. Just one nutrient deficiency may compromise the body's ability to fight cancer at the cellular level, and several nutrients are critical for maintaining healthy breast tissue.

Reference List

1. Spinella MJ, Dmitrovsky E. Aberrant retinoid signaling and breast cancer: the view from outside the nucleus. *J Natl Cancer Inst.* 2000 Mar 15;92(6):438-40.

2. Audisio M, Mastroiacovo P, Martinoli L, Fidanza A, Cappelli L, Pasquali Lasagni R, Tirelli C, Jacobelli G. Serum values of vitamins A, E, C and carotenoids in healthy adult subjects and those with breast neoplasia. *Boll Soc Ital Biol Sper.* 1989 May;65(5):473-80. Italian. PMID: 2775553.

3. Newmark HL. Vitamin D adequacy: a possible relationship to breast cancer. *Adv Exp Med Biol.* 1994;364:109-14. Review. PMID: 7725953.

4. Chen P, Li C, Li X, Li J, Chu R, Wang H. Higher dietary folate intake reduces the breast cancer risk: a systematic review and meta-analysis. *Br J Cancer.* 2014 Apr 29;110(9):2327-38. doi: 10.1038/bjc.2014.155. Epub 2014 Mar 25. Review. PMID: 24667649.

5. Liu Y, Zhou LS, Xu XM, Deng LQ, Xiao QK. Association of dietary intake of folate, vitamin B6 and B12 and MTHFR genotype with breast cancer risk. *Asian Pac J Cancer Prev.* 2013;14(9):5189-92. PMID: 24175799.

6. Zhang SM, Willett WC, Selhub J, et al. Plasma folate, vitamin B6, vitamin B12, homocysteine, and risk of breast cancer. *J Natl Cancer Inst.* 2003 Mar 5;95(5):373-80. PMID: 12618502

7. Unlü A, Ates NA, Tamer L, Ates C. Relation of glutathione S-transferase T1, M1 and P1 genotypes and breast cancer risk. *Cell Biochem Funct.* 2008 Sep-Oct;26(5):643-7. doi: 10.1002/cbf.1490. PMID: 18521819

---

8. Moradi M, Hassan Eftekhari M, Talei A, Rajaei Fard A. A comparative study of selenium concentration and glutathione peroxidase activity in normal andbreast cancer patients. *Public Health Nutr.* 2009 Jan;12(1):59-63. doi: 10.1017/S1368980008001924. Epub 2008 Mar 7. PMID: 18325137.

9. Aloia JF, Vaswani A, Yeh JK, McGowan DM, Ross P. Biochemical short-term changes produced by hormonal replacement therapy. *J Endocrinol Invest.* 1991 Dec;14(11):927-34. PMID: 1806610.

10. Abdelgawad IA, El-Mously RH, Saber MM, Mansour OA, Shouman SA. Significance of serum levels of vitamin D and some related minerals in breast cancer patients. *J Clin Exp Pathol.* 2015 Apr 1;8(4):4074-82. eCollection 2015. PMID: 26097595.

11. Ronco AL, Stefani ED, Mendoza B, Vazquez A, Abbona E, Sanchez G, Rosa AD. Mate and Tea Intake, Dietary Antioxidants and Risk of Breast Cancer: a Case-Control Study. *Asian Pac J Cancer Prev.* 2016;17(6):2923-33. PMID: 27356713.

12. Mrowicka M, Zielińska-Bliźniewska H, Pietkiewicz P, Olszewski J, Majsterek I. Evaluation of selected indicators of antioxidant status in patients with head and neck cancer. *Otolaryngol Pol.* 2015;69(5):44-50. English, Polish. PMID: 26537644.

13. Cooney RV, Dai Q, Gao YT, Chow WH, Franke AA, Shu XO, Li H, Ji B, Cai Q, Chai W, Zheng W.Low plasma coenzyme Q(10) levels and breast cancer risk in Chinese women. *Cancer Epidemiol Biomarkers Prev.* 2011 Jun;20(6):1124-30. doi: 10.1158/1055-9965.EPI-10-1261. Epub 2011 Apr 5. PMID: 21467235.

14. Szynglarewicz B, Kasprzak P, Donizy P, Biecek P, Halon A, Matkowski R. uctal carcinoma in situ on stereotactic biopsy of suspicious breast microcalcifications: Expression of SPARC (Secreted Protein, Acidic and Rich in Cysteine) can predict postoperative invasion. *J Surg Oncol.* 2016 Jul 20. doi: 10.1002/jso.24373. [Epub ahead of print] PMID: 27439354.

(Some content Adapted from SpectraCell Laboratories, Inc.)

Celiac Disease

Celiac disease is characterized by the inability to tolerate gluten, which is a protein found in wheat, rye, and barley. When a person with celiac disease ingests gluten, an allergic reaction follows that causes serious damage to the intestinal wall, ultimately creating malabsorption issues and a host of cascading health problems. Some estimate that celiac disease is prevalent in over two percent of the general population. Celiac patients are known to be at higher risk for nutrient deficiencies, largely due to malabsorption issues.[1] But when it comes to supplements, the more is better philosophy does not apply. Balance is essential.

True healing begins with the body's foundation–the vitamins, minerals, and antioxidants the body needs to function optimally every day and over a lifetime. Researchers followed a group of celiac patients who had been on a gluten-free diet for ten years and found that half of the adult celiac patients exhibited a condition of vitamin deficiency.[2] Researchers estimate that 11% to 42% of celiac patients have a Vitamin B12 deficiency that impairs function of the nervous system.[3,4] Actually, resolution of Vitamin B12 deficiency in many cases resolves neurological problems associated with celiac disease.[5]

Celiac patients are at higher risk of other B Vitamin deficiencies, specifically for folate, than others. There are several reasons for this. First, the primary transporter of folate into the bloodstream is found on the tips of the finger-like projections in the intestinal wall called *villi*. Since intestinal damage, called atrophy, is very common in celiac patients, the process of absorption of nutrients, and especially folate, is severely impaired. Second, the pH of the stomach affects folic acid absorption. The higher the pH, which indicates less acidity, of the stomach the lower the absorption of folic acid in celiac patients.[6] Third, many medications used in inflammatory conditions of the gastrointestinal tract are folate depleting.

A much higher percentage of children with celiac are deficient in magnesium, calcium, and Vitamin D compared to children without celiac. These three nutrients work together in many ways. For example, when there is sufficient Vitamin D, 30% to 45% of intestinal calcium can be absorbed. However, in the presence of Vitamin D deficiency, only 15% of calcium is absorbed, leading to

---

29

poor bone health.[7,8] A deficiency in copper often manifests as neurological problems or anemia in celiac patients. Some researchers suggest that celiac disease should be considered in patients with copper deficiency even if there are no apparent gastrointestinal problems.[9,10]

In a recent study on children with celiac disease, zinc levels were up to 30% lower in children with untreated celiac, and over 50% of patients with celiac have low zinc levels.[11,12] Since a zinc deficiency causes skin rashes, there is a likely relationship between zinc deficiencies and the skin rash experienced by some people with celiac disease. A selenium deficiency is also common in celiac patients.[13,14] Since thyroid is particularly sensitive to selenium, this deficiency can contribute to thyroid dysfunction.[15,16]

Celiac patients often experience intestinal inflammation, creating oxidative stress. This condition results in a significantly reduced antioxidant status through a depletion of glutathione, considered by many to be the most potent antioxidant in the body.[17,18] In addition, levels of other antioxidants, such as cysteine and Vitamin C, affect the glutathione status[19]. Damage from inflammation increases the permeability of the walls of the digestive tract, allowing normally benign substances into the bloodstream, where they become irritants. An allergenic, or autoimmune, response follows.[20-22]

Glutamine, an amino acid, is particularly effective in mitigating this dangerous cascade of events starting in the gut since glutamine helps to form tight junctions between cells of the delicate intestinal wall.[23,24] As might be expected, levels of carnitine, which is intimately involved in energy production, are lower in celiac patients. In fact, one study showed that fatigue was significantly reduced in a group of celiac patients when they were supplemented for six months with carnitine.[25]

Reference List

1. Guevara Pacheco G, Chávez Cortés E, Castillo-Durán C. Micronutrient deficiencies and celiac disease in Pediatrics. *Arch Argent Pediatr*. 2014 Oct;112(5):457-63. doi: 10.1590/S0325-00752014000500012. Spanish. PMID: 25192528.
2. Vici G, Belli L, Biondi M, Polzonetti V, Gluten free diet and

nutrient deficiencies: A review. *Clin Nutr.* 2016 May 7. pii: S0261-5614(16)30088-7. doi: 10.1016/j.clnu.2016.05.002. [Epub ahead of print] Review. PMID: 27211234.

3. Dickey W . Low serum vitamin B12 is common in coeliac disease and is not due to autoimmune gastritis. *Eur J Gastroenterol Hepatol.* 2002 Apr;14(4):425-7. PMID: 11943958.

4. Dahele A, Ghosh S. Vitamin B12 deficiency in untreated celiac disease. *Am J Gastroenterol.* 2001 Mar;96(3):745-50. PMID: 11280545.

5. McKeon A, Lennon VA, Pittock SJ, Kryzer TJ, Murray The neurologic significance of celiac disease biomarkers. *J. Neurology.* 2014 Nov 11;83(20):1789-96. doi: 10.1212/WNL.0000000000000970. Epub 2014 Sep 26. PMID: 25261501.

6. Santana-Porbén S, Castellanos-Fernández M. Malnutrition in adults with gastrointestinal disorders: a new reservoir of celiac disease? *Gastroenterol Mex.* 2009;74(3):202-12. Spanish. PMID: 19858008.

7. Pettifor JM. Calcium and vitamin D metabolism in children in developing countries. *Ann Nutr Metab.* 2014;64 Suppl 2:15-22. doi: 10.1159/000365124. Epub 2014 Oct 22. Review. PMID: 25341870.

8. Aloia JF, Dhaliwal R, Shieh A, Mikhail M, Fazzari M, Ragolia L, Abrams SA. Vitamin D supplementation increases calcium absorption without a threshold effect. *Am J Clin Nutr.* 2014 Mar;99(3):624-31. doi: 10.3945/ajcn.113.067199. Epub 2013 Dec 11. Erratum in: *Am J Clin Nutr.* 2014 Jul;100(1):299. PMID: 24335055.

9. Khera D, Sharma B, Singh K. Copper deficiency as a cause of neutropenia in a case of coeliac disease. *BMJ Case Rep.* 2016 Sep 15;2016. pii: bcr2016214874. doi: 10.1136/bcr-2016-214874. PMID: 27635061.

10. Patterson SK, Green PH, Tennyson CA, Lewis SK, Brannagan TH 3rd. Copper levels in patients with celiac neuropathy. *J Clin Neuromuscul Dis.* 2012 Sep;14(1):11-6. doi: 10.1097/CND.0b013e318260b455. PMID: 22922576.

11. Tran CD, Katsikeros R, Manton N, Krebs NF, Hambridge KM, Butler RN, Davidson GP. Zinc homeostasis and gut

---

function in children with celiac disease. *Am J Clin Nutr.* 2011 Oct;94(4):1026-32. doi: 10.3945/ajcn.111.018093. Epub 2011 Aug 24. PMID: 21865333.

12. Rawal P, Thapa BR, Prasad R, Prasad KK, Nain CK, Singh K. Zinc supplementation to patients with celiac disease--is it required? Rawal P, Thapa BR, Prasad R, Prasad KK, Nain CK, Singh K. *J Trop Pediatr.* 2010 Dec;56(6):391-7. doi: 10.1093/tropej/fmq011. Epub 2010 Feb 21. PMID: 20176568.

13. Kawamura T. The functional role of zinc in skin diseases. *Nihon Rinsho.* 2016 Jul;74(7):1144-9. Japanese. PMID: 27455804.

14. Ogawa Y, Kawamura T, Shimada S. Zinc and skin biology. *Arch Biochem Biophys.* 2016 Jun 7. pii: S0003-9861(16)30189-8. doi: 10.1016/j.abb.2016.06.003. [Epub ahead of print] PMID: 27288087.

15. Wu Q, Rayman MP, Lv H, Schomburg L, Cui B, et al. Low Population Selenium Status Is Associated With Increased Prevalence of Thyroid Disease. Wu Q, Rayman MP, Lv H, Schomburg L, Cui B, Gao C, Chen P, Zhuang G, Zhang Z, Peng X, Li H, Zhao Y, He X, Zeng G, Qin F, Hou P, Shi B. *J Clin Endocrinol Metab.* 2015 Nov;100(11):4037-47. doi: 10.1210/jc.2015-2222. Epub 2015 Aug 25. PMID: 26305620.

16. Schomburg L. Selenium, selenoproteins and the thyroid gland: interactions in health and disease. *Nat Rev Endocrinol.* 2011 Oct 18;8(3):160-71. doi: 10.1038/nrendo.2011.174. Review. PMID: 22009156.

17. Ward KP, Arthur JR, Russell G, Aggett PJ. Blood selenium content and glutathione peroxidase activity in children with cystic fibrosis, coeliac disease, asthma, and epilepsy. *Eur J Pediatr.* 1984 Apr;142(1):21-4. PMID: 6714254.

18. Boda M, Németh I. Decrease in the antioxidant capacity of red blood cells in children with celiac disease. *Acta Paediatr Hung.* 1992;32(3):241-55. PMID: 1476783.

19. Li C, Zhang WJ, Choi J, Frei B, Quercetin affects glutathione levels and redox ration in human aortic endothelial cells not through oxidation but formation and cellular export of quercetin-glutathione conjugates and upregulation of glutamate-cysteine ligase. *Redox Biol.* 2016 Aug 21;9:220-228. doi: 10.1016/j.redox.2016.08.012. [Epub ahead of print]

PMID: 27572418.

20. Liu Z, Li N, Neu J. Tight junctions, leaky intestines, and pediatric diseases. *Acta Paediatr.* 2005 Apr;94(4):386-93. Review. PMID: 16092447.

21. Yang PC, Wang CS, An ZY. A murine model of ulcerative colitis: induced with sinusitis-derived superantigen and food allergen. *BMC Gastroenterol.* 2005 Mar 3;5:6. Erratum in: *BMC Gastroenterol.* 2006;6:23. PMID:15745456.

22. Ghouzali I, Lemaitre C, Bahlouli W, Azhar S, Bôle-Feysot C, Meleine M, Ducrotté P, Déchelotte P, Coëffier M. Targeting immunoproteasome and glutamine supplementation prevent intestinal hyperpermeability. *Biochim Biophys Acta.* 2016 Aug 17. pii: S0304-4165(16)30291-4. doi: 10.1016/j.bbagen.2016.08.010. [Epub ahead of print] PMID: 27544233.

23. Vermeulen MA, de Jong J, Vaessen MJ, van Leeuwen PA, Houdijk AP. Glutamate reduces experimental intestinal hyperpermeability and facilitates glutamine support of gut integrity. Vermeulen MA, de Jong J, Vaessen MJ, van Leeuwen PA, Houdijk AP. *World J Gastroenterol.* 2011 Mar 28;17(12):1569-73. doi: 10.3748/wjg.v17.i12.1569. PMID: 21472123.

24. Ciacci C, Peluso G, Iannoni E, Siniscalchi M, Iovino P, Rispo A, Tortora R, Bucci C, Zingone F, Margarucci S, Calvani M. L-Carnitine in the treatment of fatigue in adult celiac disease patients: a pilot study. *Dig Liver Dis.* 2007 Oct;39(10):922-8. Epub 2007 Aug 10. PMID: 17693145.

(Some content Adapted from SpectraCell Laboratories, Inc.)

Cognitive Function

Most people want to protect their cognitive function throughout their lives. There are several micronutrients that affect this function. The B Vitamins folate, B6, and B12 are important in methylation (repairing) processes. Deficiencies in one of these vitamins can raise the homocysteine level, which is linked to increased risk of Alzheimer's disease. Vitamin B1 protects against mitochondrial dysfunction that causes dementia.[1-3] Vitamin B12 improves frontal lobe functions, such as language, especially in the elderly.[4] Choline, another member of the B-complex, is the precursor molecule for the neurotransmitter acetylcholine, which is intimately involved in memory. A choline deficiency can produce mitochondrial dysfunction in the brain that clinically presents as cognitive impairment.[6] Inositol, another member of the B Vitamins, regulates cell membrane transport, thus explaining its vital interaction with several hormone and regulatory functions. Research suggests it can protect against the formation of abnormally folded toxic proteins seen in patients with Alzheimer's disease. Inositol treatment also has beneficial effects on depression and anxiety.[7,8]

Other important vitamins include A, C, and E. In the Physician's Health Study II, Vitamin A supplementation (50 mg) improved cognition and verbal memory in men. Short-term (1 year) effects of cognitive function were not seen, but significant benefit occurred in those on long-term (18 months) treatment.[9] Next to the adrenal glands, nerve endings contain the highest levels of Vitamin C in the body. High intakes of Vitamin C are associated with lower risk of Alzheimer's disease. In addition to anti-oxidative properties, Vitamin E reduces death to cells in the hippocampus and protects the brain from glutamate toxicity. High dietary intake of Vitamin E may lower the risk of Alzheimer's.[10-12] Also, Vitamin D supplementation improves mood and cognitive function in the elderly.[13]

Several minerals are important to cognitive function. In a placebo-contolled, double blind study, chromium supplementation for twelve weeks improved cerebral function to older adults, possibly as a downstream effect of augmented glucose disposal in patients with insulin resistance.[14] Intracellular coppy deficiency increases the formation of amyloid deposits in the brain. Specifically, copper accumulates in amyloid plagues while remaining deficient in neighboring brain cells, indicating that a copper deficiency is a plausible cause of Alzheimer's.[15] When zinc does not function as expected, there is a negative alteration of the immune-inflammatory system. This deficiency may cause depression, impair learning and memory, and reduce neurogenesis. Zinc also regulates the plasticity of the synapses.[16-18] Iron supplementation helps to prevent mitochondria decay in aging.[19]

The amino acid carnitine with its potent antioxidant properties has a role in the transport of fatty acid to the mitochondria, explaining its beneficial effects on both physical and mental fatigue. Several studies have demonstrated a consistent improvement in memory, focus, and cognition with carnitine supplementation.[20,21] The antioxidant glutathione is consumed faster in brain tissue in the presence of choline deficiency. The amino acids glutamine and asparagine function as neurotransmitters in the brain, so are important. The amino acid serine is the major component of phosphatidylserine, an integral part of cell membranes in the brain. Phosphatidylserine increases the release of several neurotransmitters, including dopamine, serotonin, acetylcholine, and epinephrine, thus improving the rate at which mental processes occur, but without the hyperactivity or compulsive behavior that often occurs with drugs that stimulate a single neurotransmitter.[22]

Finally, oleic acid, a fatty acid found primarily in olive oil and the precursor to oleamide, interacts with several neurotransmitters and has demonstrated antidepressant-like properties. Oleic acid also aids the absorption of Vitamin A into cells.[23-24] Research clearly indicates that lipoic acid is a potent neuroprotective antioxidant that strengthens memory and stimulates nerve growth as well as protecting against the neuronal injury that occurs in the presences of toxic proteins in the brain tissue of Alzheimer's patients.[25-26]

Reference List

1. Kim JM, Stewart R, Kim SW, et al. Changes in folate, vitamin B12 and homocysteine associated with incident dementia. *J Neurol Neurosurg Psychiatry* 2008;79:864-868.
2. D'Anci KE, Rosenberg IH. Folate and brain function in the elderly. *Curr Opin Clin Nutr Metab Care* 2004;7:659-664.
3. Smith AD, Smith SM, de Jager CA, et al. Homocysteine-lowering by B vitamins slows the rate of accelerated brain

atrophy in mild cognitive impairment: a randomized controlled trial. *PLoS One* 2010;5:e12244.

4. Clarke R, Birks J, Nexo E, et al. Low vitamin B-12 status and risk of cognitive decline in older adults. *Am J Clin Nutr* 2007;86:1384-1391.

5. Troen AM, Chao WH, Crivello NA, et al. Cognitive impairment in folate-deficient rats corresponds to depleted brain phosphatidylcholine and is prevented by dietary methionine without lowering plasma homocysteine. *J Nutr* 2008;138:2502-2509.

6. Pacelli C, Coluccia A, Grattagliano I, et al. Dietary choline deprivation impairs rat brain mitochondrial function and behavioral phenotype. *J Nutr* 2010;140:1072-1029.

7. Choi JK, Carreras I, Dedeoglu A, Jenkins BG, et al. Detection of increased scyllo-inositol in brain with magnetic resonance spectroscopy after dietary supplementation in Alzheimer's disease mouse models. *Neuropharmacology* 2010;59:353-357.

8. Coupland NJ, Ogilvie CJ, Hegadoren KM, et al. Decreased prefrontal Myo-inositol in major depressive disorder. *Biol Psychiatry* 2005;57:1526-1534.

9. Grodstein F, Kang JH, Glynn RJ, et al. A randomized trial of beta carotene supplementation and cognitive function in men: the Physicians' Health Study II. *Arch Int Med 2007*; 167:2184-2190.23.

10. Bourre JM. Effects of nutrients (in food) on the structure and function of the nervous system: update on dietary requirements for brain. Part 1: micronutrients. *J Nutr Health Aging* 2006;10:377-385.

11. Kidd PM. A review of nutrients and botanicals in the integrative management of cognitive dysfunction. Alt Med Rev 1999;4:144-161.

12. Engelhart MJ, Geerlings MI, Ruitenberg A, et al. Dietary intake of antioxidants and risk of Alzheimer disease. *JAMA* 2002;287:3223-3229.

13. Wilkins CH, et al. Vitamin D deficiency is associated with low mood and worse cognitive performance in older adults. *Am J Geriatr Psychiatry*2006;14:1032-1040

14. Krikorian R, Eliassen JC, Boespfluget EL, et al. Improved cognitive-cerebral function in older adults with chromium

supplementation. *Nutr Neurosci* 2010;13:116-122.

15. Cater MA, McInnes KT, Li QX, et al. Intracellular Copper Deficiency Increases Amyloid-beta Secretion by Diverse Mechanisms. *Biochem J* 2008;412:141-152.

16. Tupe RP, Chiplonkar SA, et al. Zinc supplementation improved cognitive performance and taste acuity in Indian adolescent girls. *J Am Coll Nutr* 2009;28:388-396.

17. Szewyzck, Kubera M, Nowak G, et al. The role of zinc in neurodegenerative inflammatory pathways in depression. *Prog Neuropsychopharmacol Biol Psychiatry* 2011;35;693-701.

18. Prasad AS. Impact of the discovery of human zinc deficiency on health. *J Am Coll Nutr* 2009;28:257-265.

19. Atamna H. Heme, iron, and the mitochondrial decay of ageing. *Ageing Res Rev* 2004;3:303-318.

20. Malaguarnera M, Gargante MP, Cristaldi E, et al. Acetyl L-carnitine (ALC) treatment in elderly patients with fatigue. *Arch Gerontol Geriatr* 2008;46:181-190.

21. Malaguarnera M, Vacante M, Avitabileet T, et al. L-Carnitine treatment reduces severity of physical and mental fatigue and increases cognitive functions in centenarians: a randomized and controlled clinical trial. *Am J Clin Nutr* 2007;86:1738-1744.

22. Moreno-Fuenmayor H, Borjas L, Arrieta A, Valera V, Socorro-Candanoza L, et al. Plasma excitatory amino acids in autism. *Invest Clin* 1996;37:113-128.

23. Raju M, Lakshminarayana R, Krishnakantha TP, Baskaran V, et al. Micellar oleic and eicosapentaenoic acid but not linoleic acid influences the beta-carotene uptake and its cleavage into retinol in rats. *Mol Cell Biochem* 2006;288:7-15.

24. Akanmu MA, Adeosun SO, Ilesanmi OR, et al. Neuropharmacological effects of oleamide in male and female mice. *Behav Brain Res* 2007;182:88-94.

25. Cho JY, Hyun SU, Eun B, et al. The combination of exercise training and alpha-lipoic acid treatment has therapeutic effects on the pathogenic phenotypes of Alzheimer's disease in NSE/APPsw-transgenic mice. *Int J Mol Med* 2010;25:337-346.

26. Manda K, Ueno M, Moritake T, Anzai K. Radiation-induced

cognitive dysfunction and cerebellar oxidative stress in mice: protective effect of alpha-lipoic acid. *Behav Brain Res* 2007;177:7-14.

(Some content Adapted from SpectraCell Laboratories, Inc.)

Depression

Since WWII, the diagnosis of depression has continued to rise. Recent studies suggest that most anti-depressant drugs are not effective for the broad spectrum of depression.[1] The increased complaint of depression and the low effectiveness of antidepressants suggest a need to explore other avenues for handling this condition. There are several B Vitamins that affect depression. For example, folate is the building block for many feel-good neurotransmitters, such as serotonin, dopamine and norepinephrine. Low folate causes a poor response to antidepressant medications. The lower the folate the more severe the depression.[2-5] Depression may also be a manifestation of Vitamin B12 deficiency because repletion of B12 to adequate levels can improve treatment response. A B12 deficiency is common in psychiatric disorders.[6-8] Vitamin B6 is a cofactor for serotonin and dopamine production. Studies indicate that low levels may predispose people to depression.[9-11]

A Vitamin B2 deficiency has been implicated in depression due to its role in methylation reactions in the brain.[12,13] Inositol, another B Vitamin, influences signaling processes in the brain. It is particularly effective in SSRI (selective serotonin reuptake inhibitor) sensitive disorders.[14,15] A deficiency in the B Vitamin biotin has induced depression in animal and human studies.[16,17] Another major vitamin that plays a role is Vitamin D. Clinical trials with Vitamin D suggest that increasing blood levels of Vitamin D, which is actually a hormone precursor, may improve symptoms of depression.[18-20]

Deficiencies in minerals also effect depression. Magnesium deficiency damages NMDA (N-methyl-D-aspartate) receptors in the brain that regulate mood. It also has well-documented anti-depressant effects.[21,22] Selenium is an integral part of regulatory proteins, called selenoproteins, in the brain. Supplementation trials are promising. Selenium also may alleviate postpartum depression.[25,26] Zinc improves efficacy of antidepressant drugs. It is particularly useful for treatment resistant patients. It regulates many neurotransmitters.[27-30] Chromium elevates serotonin (feel-good neurotransmitter) levels in the brain. It may be particularly effective for eating symptoms of depression, such as carbohydrate craving and increased appetite, due to its effect on blood sugar regulation.[31,32]

Some amino acids and anitoxidants aid in preventing depression. Carnitine increases serotonin and noradrenaline, which

41

lift mood. In trials, carnitine alleviated depression with few, if any, side effects.[34,35] Serine regulates brain chemistry. It is involved in NMDA receptor function and acts as a neurotransmitter. Low levels correlate with the severity of depression.[39,40] Oxidative stress in the brain alters neurotransmitter function. Antioxidants protect the brain, which is very sensitive to oxidation. Several antioxidants—Vitamins A, C and E, lipoic acid, CoQ10, glutathione and cysteine—play a key role in prevention and treatment of depression.[36-38]

Reference List

1. Insel T. *Director's blog: Antidrepressants: A complicated picture.* National Institute of Mental Health. http://www.nimh.nih.gov/about/director/2011/antidepressants-a-complicated-picture.shtml. Dec 2016. Accessed 13 Sep 2016.
2. Coppen A, Bailey J. Enhancement of the antidepressant action of fluoxetine by folic acid: a randomized, placebo controlled trial. *J Affect Disord* 2000;60:121-130.
3. Miller A. The methylation, neurotransmitter and antioxidant connections between folate and depression. *Altern Med Rev* 2008;13:216-226.
4. Papakostas G, Petersen T, Mischoulon D, et al. Serum folate, vitamin B12, and homocysteine in major depressive disorder, Part 1: predictors of clinical response in fluoxetine-resistant depression. *J Clin Psychiatry* 2004;65:1090-1095.
5. Wesson V, Levitt A, Joffe R. Change in folate status with antidepressant treatment.
6. Kate N, Grover S, Agarwal M. Does B12 deficiency lead to a lack of treatment response to conventional antidepressants? *Psychiatry* 2010;7:42-44
7. Hintikka J, Tolmunen T, Tanskanen A, et al. High vitamin B12 level and good treatment outcome may be associated in major depressive disorder. *BMC Psychiatry* 2003:3:17.
8. Bhat A, Srinivasan K, Kurpad S, et al. Psychiatric presentations of vitamin B12 deficiency. *J of Indian Med Ass* 2007;105:395-396.
9. Elders, Falcon L, Tucker K. Vitamin B6 is associated with depressive symptomatology in Massachusetts. *J Am Coll Nutr* 2008;27:421-427.
10. William A, Cotter A, Sabina A, et al. The role for vitamin B-6

---

as treatment for depression: a systematic review. *Fam Pract* 2005;22:532-537.

11. Hvas A, Juul S, Bech P, et al. Vitamin B6 level is associated with symptoms of depression. *Psychother Psychosom* 2004;73:340-343.

12. Miyake Y, Sasaki S, Tanaka K, et al. Dietary folate and vitamins B12, B6 and B2 intake and the risk of postpartum depression in Japan: the Osaka Maternal and Child Health Study. *J Affect Disord* 2006;96:133-138.

13. Bell I, Morrow F, Read M, et al. Low thyroxine levels in female psychiatric in patients with riboflavin deficiency: implications for folate-dependent methylation. *Acta Psychiatr Scand* 1992;85:360-363.

14. Levine J, Barak Y, Gonzalves M, et al. Double-blind, controlled trial of inositol treatment of depression. *Am J Psychiatry* 1995;152:792-794.

15. Brink C, Viljoen S, de Kock S, et al. Effects of myo-inositol versus fluoxetine and imipramine pretreatments on serotonin 5HT2A and muscarinic acetylcholine receptors in human neuroblastoma cells. *Metab Brain Dis* 2004;19:51-70.

16. Levenson J. Biotin-responsive depression during hyperalimentation. *J Parenter Enteral Nutr* 1983;7:181-183.

17. Osada K, Komai M, et al. Experimental study of fatigue provoked by biotin deficiency in mice. *Int J Vitam Nutr Res* 2004;74:334-340.

18. Jorde R, Sneve M, Figenschau Y, et al. Effects of vitamin D supplementation on symptoms of depression in overweight and obese subjects: randomized double blind trial. *J Intern Med* 2008;264:599-609.

19. Högberg G, Gustafsson SA, Hällström T, et al. Depressed adolescents in a case-series were low in vitamin D and depression was ameliorated by vitamin D supplementation. *Acta Paediatr* 2012;101:779-783.

20. Berk M, Sanders K, Pasco J, et al. Vitamin D deficiency may play a role in depression. *Med Hypotheses* 2007;69:1316-1319.

21. Nechifor M. Magnesium in major depression. *Magnes Res* 2009;22:163S-166S.

22. Eby G, Eby K. Magnesium for treatment-resistant depression: a review and hypothesis. *Med Hypotheses* 2010;74:649-660.

23. Szewezyk B, Poleszak E, Sowa-Kuema M, et al. Antidepressant

activity of zinc and magnesium in view of the current hypotheses of antidepressant action. *Pharmacol Rep* 2008;60:588-589.

24. Eby G, Eby K. Rapid recovery from major depression using magnesium treatment. *Med Hypotheses* 2006;67:362-70.

25. Mokhber N, Namjoo M, Tara F, et al. Effect of supplementation with selenium on postpartum depression: a randomized double-blind placebo-controlled trial. *J Matern Fetal Neonatal Med* 2011;24:104-108.

26. Benton D, Cook R. The impact of selenium supplementation on mood. *Biol Psychiatry* 1991;29:1092-1098.

27. Smeland O, Meisingset T, Borges K, et al. Chronic acetyl-L-carnitine alters brain energy metabolism and increases noradrenaline and serotonin content in healthy mice. *Neurochem Int* 2012;61:100-107.

28. Garzya G, Corallo D, Fiore A, et al. Evaluation of the effects of L-acetylcarnitine on senile patients suffering from depression. *Drugs Exp Clin Res* 1990;16:101-106.

29. Cope E, Levenson C. Role of zinc in the development and treatment of mood disorders. *Curr Opin Clin Nutr Metab Care* 2010;13:685-689.

30. Nowak G, Siwek M, Dudek D, et al. Effect of zinc supplementation on antidepressant therapy in unipolar depression: a preliminary placebo-controlled study. *Pol J Pharmacol* 2003;55:1143-1147.

31. Maes M, Vandoolaeghe E, Neels H, et al. Lower serum zinc in major depression is a sensitive marker of treatment resistance and of the immune/inflammatory response in that illness. *Psychiatry* 1997;42:349-358.

32. Levenson C. Zinc, the new antidepressant? *Nutr Rev* 2006;64:39-42.

33. Attenburrow M, Odontiadis J, Murray B, et al. Chromium treatment decreases the sensitivity of 5-HT2A receptors. *Pychopharmacology* 2002;159:432-436.

34. Docherty J, Sack D, Roffman M, et al. A double-blind, placebo-controlled, exploratory trial of chromium picolinate in atypical depression: effect on carbohydrate craving. *J Psychiatr Pract* 2005;11:302-314.

35. Davidson J, Abraham K, Connor K, et al. Effectiveness of chromium in atypical depression: a placebo controlled trial. *Biol Psychiatry* 2003;53:261-264.

---

36. Bodnar L, Wisner K. Nutrition and depression: Implications for improving mental health among child-bearing-aged women. *Biol Psychiatry* 2005;58:679-685.
37. Maes M, Mihaylova I, Kubera M, et al. Lower plasma Coenzyme Q10 in depression: a marker for treatment resistance and chronic fatigue in depression and a risk factor to cardiovascular disorder in that illness. *Neuro Endocrinol Lett* 2009;30:462-469.
38. Tsuboi H, Shimoi K, Kinae N, et al. Depressive symptoms are independently correlated with lipid peroxidation in a female population: comparison with vitamins and carotenoids. *J Psychosom Res* 2004;56:53-58.
39. de Koning T, Klomp L. Serine-deficiency syndromes. *Curr Opin Neurol* 2004;17:197-204.
40. Mitani H, Shirayama Y, Yamada T, et al. Correlation between plasma levels of glutamate, alanine and serine with severity of depression. *Prog Neuropsychopharmacol Biol Psychiatry* 2006;30:1155-1158.

Additional references at **http://www.spectracell.com/online-library-mnt-depression-abstract**.

(Some content Adapted from SpectraCell Laboratories, Inc.)

Diabetes

Diabetes, a relatively unknown condition in the mid twentieth century, has unexpectedly expanded to include almost 10% of the U.S. population and 8.5% of the global population.[1] Several important vitamins support the prevention of diabetes. Vitamin B12 deficiency is common in diabetics because metformin, a diabetes medication, depletes B12.[2,3] Vitamin B3 preserves B-cell function in type 1 diabetics. It is part of GTF (glucose tolerance factor) that facilitates insulin binding.[4-6] Vitamin D lowers the risk of type 1 and 2 diabetes: It suppresses inflammation of pancreatic B-cells. Vitamin D receptor gene variant is linked to diabetes.[7-9] Vitamin E confers protection against diabetes by protecting pancreatic B-cells from oxidative stress induced damage. Vitamin E may prevent progression of type I diabetes.[7-10]

Vitamin C lowers glycosylated hemoglobin (HbA1c) and fasting and post-meal glucose levels in type 2 diabetics.[11-13] Evidence suggests that the B Vitamin inositol may be effective in treating diabetic neuropathy.[14,15] Biotin stimulates glucose-induced insulin secretion in pancreatic B-cells. High doses of biotin can improve glycemic control in diabetics.[16-18]

Several minerals assist the prevention of diabetes. Zinc is needed in the synthesis, storage, and secretion of insulin. It protects pancreatic B-cells from damage. It affects the expression of genes linked to diabetes.[19,20] Magnesium reduces insulin sensitivity. Low magnesium exacerbates foot ulcers in diabetics.[21,22] Chromium helps insulin attach to a cell's receptors increasing glucose uptake into the cell. A chromium deficiency can cause insulin resistance. Supplementation studies show dose-dependent benefits for type II diabetics, meaning the effects change as the dose changes.[23-25]

Finally, there are amino acids, co-enzymes, and antioxidants that are key to understanding diabetes. The amino acid carnitine reduces and even prevents pain from diabetic neuropathy. It improves insulin sensitivity by increasing glucose uptake and storage.[26-29] Glutamine stimulates a hormone called GLP-1 (glucagon-like peptide 1) that regulates insulin secretion after meals. It improves *insulin signaling* (the mechanisms involved in biologic responses to insulin) and sensitivity.[30,31] Coenzyme Q10 protects the kidneys from diabetes related damage because it improves glycemic control in type 2 diabetics.[32,33] Glutathione-containing enzymes protect B-cells, cells that are particularly sensitive to oxidative stress. Type 2 diabetics have abnormal antioxidant status of increased oxidative stress. Supplementation with the glutathione precursor cysteine restores antioxidant status.[34-36] Lipoic acid heightens glucose uptake in skeletal muscle tissue and improves glucose tolerance in type 2 diabetics. It is a very effective treatment for diabetic neuropathy.[37-39]

Reference List

1. World Health Organization. *Diabetes Fact Sheet.* http://www.who.int/mediacentre/factsheets/fs312/en/. 2016. Accessed 13 Sep 2016.
2. Pflipsen M, Oh R, Saguil A, et al. The prevalence of vitamin B(12) deficiency in patients with type 2 diabetes: a cross-sectional study. *J Am Board Fam Med* 2009;22:528-534.
3. Wulffele M, Kooy A, Lehert P, et al. Effects of short-term treatment with metformin on serum concentrations of homocysteine, folate and vitamin B12 in type 2 diabetes mellitus: a randomized, placebo-controlled trial. *J InternMed* 2003;254:455-463.
4. Pozzilli P, Browne P, Kolb H. Meta-analysis of nicotinamide treatment in patients with recent-onset IDDM. The Nicotinamide Trialists. *Diabetes Care* 1996;19:1357-1363.
5. Greenbaum C, Kahn S, Palmer J. Nicotinamide's effects on glucose metabolism in subjects at risk for IDDM. *Diabetes* 1996;45:1631-1634.
6. Visalli N, Cavallo M, Signore A, et al. A multicentre randomized trial of two different doses of nicotinamide in patients with recent-onset type 1 diabetes (the IMDIAB VI). *Diabetes Metab Res Rev* 1999;15:181-185.
7. Hypponene E. Micronutrients and the risk of type 1 diabetes: vitamin D, vitamin E and nicotinamide. *Nutr Rev* 2004;62:340-347.
8. Liu E, Meigs J, Pittas A, et al. Plasma 25-hydroxyvitamin d is associated with markers of the insulin resistance phenotype in nondiabetic adults. *J Nutr* 2009;139:329-334.
9. Bailey R, Cooper J, Zeitels L, et al. Association of the vitamin D metabolism gene CYP27B1 with type 1 diabetes. *Diabetes* 2007;56:2616-2621.

10. Knekt P, Reunanen A, Marniemi J, et al. Low vitamin E status is a potential risk factor for insulin-dependent diabetes mellitus. *J Intern Med* 1999;245:99-102.
11. Dakhale G, Chaudhari H, et al. Supplementation of vitamin C reduces blood glucose and improves glycosylated hemoglobin in type 2 diabetes mellitus: a randomized, double-blind study. *Adv Pharmacol Sci* 2011;195271.
12. Afkhami-Ardekani M, Shojaoddiny-Ardekani A. Effect of vitamin C on blood glucose, serum lipids and serum insulin in type 2 diabetes patients. *Indian J Med Res* 2007;126:471-474.
13. Yamada H, Yamada K, Waki M, et al. Lymphocyte and plasma vitamin C levels in type II diabetic patients with and without diabetes complications. *Diabetes Care* 2004;27:2491-2492.
14. Farias V, Macedo F, Oquendo M, et al. Chronic treatment with D-chiro-inositol prevents autonomic and somatic neuropathy in STZ-induced diabetic mice. *Diabetes Obes Metab* 2011;13:243-250.
15. Sima A, Dunlap J, Davidson E, et al. Supplemental myo-inositol precents L-fucose-induced diabetic neuropathy. *Diabetes* 1997;46:301-306.
16. Albarracin C, Fuqua B, Evans J, et al. Chromium picolinate and biotin combination improves glucose metabolism in treated, uncontrolled overweight to obese patients with type 2 diabetes. *Diabetes Metab Res Rev* 2008;24:41-51.
17. Furukawa Y. Enhancement of glucose-induced insulin secretion and modification of glucose metabolism by biotin. *Nippon Rinsho* 1999;57:2261-2269.
18. Larrieta E, de la Vega-Monroy M, Vital P, et al. Effects of biotin deficiency on pancreatic islet morphology, insulin sensitivity and glucose homeostatis. *J Nutr Biochem* 2012;23:392-399.
19. Jansen J, Karges W, Rink L. Zinc and diabetes – clinical links and molecular mechanisms. *J Nutr Biochem* 2009;20:399-417.
20. Sun Q, van Dam R, Willett W, et al. A prospective study of zinc intake and risk of type 2 diabetes in women. *Diabetes Care* 2009;32:629-634.
21. Takaya J, Higashino H, Kobayashi Y. Intracellular

---

magnesium and insulin resistance. *Magnes Res* 2004;17:126-136.

22. Rodriguez-Moran M, Guerrero-Romero F. Low serum magnesium levels and foot ulcers in subjects with type 2 diabetes. *Arch Med Res* 2001;34:300-303.

23. Broadhurst C, Domenico P. Clinical studies on chromium picolinate supplementation in diabetes mellitus—a review. *Diabetes Technol Ther* 2006;8:677-687.

24. Hua Y, Clark S, Ren J, et al. Molecular mechanisms of chromium in alleviating insulin resistance. *J Nutr Biochem* 2012;23:313-319.

25. Cefalu W, Rood J, Pinsonat P, et al. Characterization of the metabolic and physiologic response to chromium supplementation in subjects with type 2 diabetes mellitus. *Metabolism* 2010;59:755-762.

26. Mingrone G, Greco A, Capristo E, et al. L-carnitine improves glucose disposal in type 2 diabetic patients. *J Am Coll Nutr* 1999;18:77-82.

27. Molfino A, Cascino A, Conte C. Caloric restriction and L-carnitine administration improves insulin sensitivity in patients with impaired glucose metabolism. *J Parenter Enteral Nutr* 2010;34:295-299.

28. Sima A. Acetyl-L-carnitine improves pain, nerve regeneration, and vibratory perception in patients with chronic diabetic neuropathy: an analysis of two randomized placebo-controlled trials. *Diabetes Care* 2005;28:89-94.

29. Sima A. Acetyl-L-carnitine in diabetic polyneuropathy: experimental and clinical data. *CNS Drugs* 2007;21 Suppl 1:13-23.

30. Greenfield J, Farooqi I, Keogh J, et al. Oral glutamine increases circulating glucagon-like peptide 1, glucagon, and insulin concentrations in lean, obese, and type 2 diabetic subjects. *Am J Clin Nutr* 2009;89:106-113.

31. Reimann F, Williams L, da Silva Xavier G, et al. Glutamine potently stimulates glucagon-like peptide-1 secretion from GLUTag cells. *Diabetologia* 2004;47:1592-1601.

32. Sourris K, Harcourt B, Tang P, et al. Ubiquinone (coenzyme Q10) prevents renal mitochondrial dysfunction in an experimental model of type 2 diabetes. *Free Radic Biol Med* 2012;52:716-723.

---

33. Mezawa M, Takemoto M, Onishi S, et al. The reduced form of coenzyme Q10 improves glycemic control in patients with type 2 diabetes: An open label pilot study. *Biofactors* 2012 [Epub ahead of print].
34. Newsholme P, Rebelato E, Abdulkader F, et al. Reactive oxygen and nitrogen species generation, antioxidant defenses, and β-cell function: a critical role for amino acids. *J Clin Endocrinol* 2012;214:11-20.
35. De Mattia G, Bravi M, Laurenti O, et al. Influence of reduced glutathione infusion on glucose metabolism in patients with non-insulin-dependent diabetes mellitus. *Metabolism* 1998;47:993-997.
36. Sekhar R, Patel S, Guthikonda A, et al. Deficient synthesis of glutathione underlies oxidative stress in aging and can be corrected by dietary cysteine and glycine supplementation. *Am J Clin Nutr* 2011;94:847-853.
37. Porasuphatana S, Suddee S, Nartnampong A, et al. Glycemic and oxidative status of patients with type 2 diabetes mellitus following oral administration of alpha-lipoic acid: a randomized double-blinded placebo-controlled study. *Asia Pac J Clin Nutr* 2012;21:12-21.
38. Ziegler D, Ametov A, Barinov A, et al. Oral treatment with alpha-lipoic acid improves symptomatic diabetic polyneuropathy: the SYDNEY 2 trial. *Diabetes Care* 2006;29:2365-2370.
39. Ansar H, Mazloom Z, Kazemi F, et al. Effect of alpha-lipoic acid on blood glucose, insulin resistance and glutathione peroxidase of type 2 diabetic patients. *Saudi Med J* 2011;32:584-588.

Additional references at http://www.spectracell.com/online-library-mnt-diabetes-abstract
(Some content Adapted from SpectraCell Laboratories, Inc.)

Dyslipidemia (Abnormal Cholesterol or Triglycerides)

Dyslipidemia, the elevation of plasma cholesterol/triglycerides or a low high-density lipoprotein level, contributes to the development of artherosclerosis. There are several vitamins important to regulating dyslipidemia. Vitamin C protects LDL (low density lipoprotein) from oxidation, thus making it less "sticky" and prone to atherosclerosis (clogging of arteries). It prevents white blood cells (monocytes) and oxidized LDL from sticking to blood vessel wall. It lowers Lp(a) (a lipoprotein subclass) in some people.[1-3] Vitamin D suppresses foam cell formation, thus reducing risk of lipid-related arterial blockages.

There are some vitamin deficiencies specifically linked to dyslipidemia.[4,5] Vitamin B3 (niacin) effectively lowers the highly atherogenic Lp(a) by decreasing its rate of synthesis in the liver.[6,7] Vitamin B5 (pantothenic acid) favorably alters low-density lipoprotein metabolism and reduces triglycerides. The full benefit of lipid lowering effects may not be seen for up to four months, however.[8,9] Inositol decreases small dense LDL especially in patients with metabolic syndrome. It also lowers triglycerides.[10-12] Choline regulates HDL metabolism and is part of the enzyme lecithin-cholesterol acyltransferase (a transfer enzyme) that has a major impact on the metabolism of lipoprotein.[13,14]

Several minerals are also important to regulating cholesterol/triglycerides. Manganese is a cofactor to the antioxidant superoxide dismutase that repairs damage to the blood vessels caused by oxidized LDL.[15,16] While a magnesium deficiency causes pro-atherogenic (heart-disease causing) changes in lipoprotein metabolism, magnesium protects LDL from being oxidized.[17,18] Chromium improves the dyslipidemia that co-occurs with insulin resistance. It may increase HDL (high density lipoprotein) and has a synergistic effect with niacin (B3) for dyslipidemia.[19-21] Several copper-dependent enzymes affect lipoprotein metabolism, and a deficiency contributes to the fatty buildup in arteries caused by dyslipidemia.[22-24]

The trace mineral selenium prevents post-prandial (after a meal) changes in lipoproteins that make them susceptible to oxidation and, thus, harmful.[25,26] Finally, suboptimal zinc raises dangerous lipoproteins that promote vascular formation. Cellular zinc controls the gene that makes heart-protective HDL.[27-29]

53

The amino acid carnitine and two antioxidants also can help. In carnitine supplementation studies, carnitine lowers triglycerides, oxidized LDL, and the atherogenic Lp(a). This effect is likely due to its role in transporting fatty acids into cells so they can be used as fuel.[30-32] Lipoic acid improves lipid profiles by reducing small, dense LDL (dangerous type). It also protects the vascular lining from oxidized cholesterol.[33] Statins, often prescribed for dyslipidemia, deplete CoQ10, which lowers Lp(a) and improves effectiveness of some dyslipidemia meds.[34,35]

Reference List

1. Woolard K, Loryman C, Merith E, et al. Effects of vitamin C on monocyte: endothelial cell adhesion in healthy subjects. *Biochem Biophys Res Commun* 2002;294:1161-1168.
2. Shariat S, Mostafavi S, Khackpour F. Antioxidant effects of Vitamin C and E on the low density lipoprotein oxidation mediated by myeloperoxidase. *Iran Biomed J* 2013;17:22-28.
3. Rath M. Lipoprotein-a reduction by ascorbate. *J Orthomolec Med* 1992;7:81-82.
4. Riek A, Oh J, Bernal-Mizrachi C. Vitamin D regulates macrophage cholesterol metabolism in diabetes. *J Steroid Biochem Mol Biol* 2010;121:430-433.
5. Guasch A, Bulló M, Rabassa A, et al. Plasma vitamin D and parathormone are associated with obesity and atherogenic dyslipidemia: a cross-sectional study. *Cardiovasc Diabeto.* 2012;11:149.
6. Seed M, O'Connor B, Perombolelon N, et al. The effect of nicotinic acid and acipimox on lipoprotein(a) concentration and turnover. *Atherosclerosis* 1993;101:61-68.
7. Kostner K, Gupta S. Niacin: a lipid polypill? *Expert Opin Pharmacother* 2008;9:2911-20.
8. Rumberger J, Napolitano J, Azmumano I, et al. Pantethine, a derivative of vitamin B(5) used as a nutritional supplement, favorably alters low-density lipoprotein cholesterol metabolism in low- to moderate-cardiovascular risk North American subjects: a triple-blinded placebo and diet-controlled investigation. *Nutr Res* 2011;31:608-615.
9. McRae M, Treatment of hyperlipoproteinemia with pantethine: a review and analysis of efficacy and tolerability.

Nutr Res 2005; 25:319-333.

10. Maeba R, Hara H, Ishikawa H, et al. Myo-inositol treatment increases serum plasmalogens and decreases small dense LDL, particularly in hyperlipidemic subjects with metabolic syndrome. *J Nutr Sci Vitaminol* 2008;54:196-202.

11. Jariwalla R. Inositol hexaphosphate (IP6) as an anti-neoplastic and lipid-lowering agent. *Anticancer Res* 1999;19:3699-702.

12. Minnozzi M, Nordio M, Pajalich R. The Combined therapy myo-inositaol plus D-Chiro-inositol, in a physiological ratio, reduces the cardiovascular risk by improving the lipid profile in PCOS patients. *Eur Rev Med Pharmacol Sci* 2013;17:537-40.

13. Kunnen S, Van Eck M. Lecithin: cholesterol acyltransferase: old friend or foe in atherosclerosis? *J Lipid Res* 2012;53:1783-99.

14. Vance D. Role of phosphatidylcholine biosynthesis in the regulation of lipoprotein homeostasis. *Curr Opin Lipidol* 200819:229-34.

15. Takabe W, Li R, Ai L, et al. Oxidized low-density lipoprotein-activated c-Jun NH2-terminal kinase regulates manganese superoxide dismutase ubiquitination: implication for mitochondrial redox status and apoptosis. *Arteriosler Thromb Vasc Biol.* 2010; 30: 436-461.

16. Perrotta I, Perrotta E, Sesti S, et al. MnSOD expression in human atherosclerotic plaques: an immunohistochemical and ultrastructural study. *Cardiovasc Pathol* 2013;Epub ahead of print.

17. Maier J. Low magnesium and atherosclerosis: an evidence-based link. *Mol Aspects Med* 2003;24:137- 146.

18. Sherer Y, Bitzur R, Cohen H, et al. Mechanisms of action of the anti-atherogenic effect of magnesium: lessons from a mouse model. *Magnes Res* 2001;14:173-179.

19. Sundaram B, Singhal K, Sandhir R. Anti-atherogenic effect of chromium picolinate in streptozotocin-induced experimental diabetes. *J Diabetes* 2013;5:43-50.

20. Sealls W, Penque B, Elmendorf J. Evidence that chromium modulates cellular cholesterol homeostasis and ABCA1 functionality impaired by hyperinsulinemia--brief report. *Arterioscler Thromb Vasc Biol* 2011;31:139-40.

21. Press R, Geller J, Evans G. The effect of chromium picolinate on serum cholesterol and apolpoprtoein farctions in human subjects. *West J Med.* 1990;152:41-5.
22. Hamilton I, Gilmore W, Starin J. Marginal copper deficiency and atherosclerosis. *Biol Trace Elem Res* 200;78:179-87.
23. DiSilvestro R, Joseph E, Zhang W, et al. A randomized trial of copper supplementation effect on blood copper enzyme activities and parameters related to cardiovascular health. *Metabolism* 2012;61:1242-6.
24. Natella F, Fidale M, Tubaro F, et al. Selenium supplementation prevents the increase in atherogenic electronegative LDL (LDL minus) in the postprandial phase. *Nutr Metab Cardiovasc Dis* 2007;17:649-56.
25. Kaur H, Bansal M. Studies on scavenger receptors under experimental hypercholesterolemia: modulation on selenium supplementation. *Biol Trace Elem Res* 2011;143:310-9.
26. Beattie J, Gordon M, Duthie S, et al. Suboptimal dietary zinc intake promotes vascular Inflammation and atherogenesis in a mouse model of atherosclerosis. *Mol Nutr Food Res* 2012;56:1097-1105.
27. Wu J, Wu Y, Reaves S, et al. Apolipoprotein A-I gene expression is regulated by cellular zinc status in hepG2 cells. *Am J Physiol.* 1999;277:C537-44.
28. Shen H, MacDonald R, Bruemmer D, et al. Zinc deficiency alters lipid metabolism in LDL receptor deficient mice treated with rosiglitazone. *J Nutr* 2007;137:2339-45.
29. Malaguarnera M, Vacante M, Avitabile T, et al. L-Carnitine supplementation reduces oxidized LDL cholesterol in patients with diabetes. *Am J Clin Nutr* 2009;89:71-76.
30. Sirtori C, Calabresi L, Ferrara S, et al. L-carnitine reduces plasma lipoprotein(a) levels in patients with hyper Lp(a). *Nutr Metab Cardiovasc Dis* 2000;10:247-251.
31. Derosa G, Cicera A, Gaddi A, et al. The effect of l-carnitine on lipoprotein(a) levels in hyper-cholesterolemic patients with type 2 diabetes mellitus. *Clin Ther* 2003; 25:1429-1439.
32. Zhang Y, Han P, Wu N, et al. Amelioration of Lipid Abnormalities by A-Lipoic acid Through Antioxidative and Anti-inflammatory Effects. *Obesity* 2011; 19:116-117.
33. Harding S, Rideout T, Jones P. Evidence for using alpha-lipoic acid in reducing lipoprotein and inflammatory related

cardiovascular risk. *J of Dietary Suppl* 2012;9:116-127.
34. Langsjoen P, Langsjoen A. The clinical use of HMG CoA-reductase inhibitors and the associated depletion of Coenzyme Q10. A review of animal and human publications. *Biofactors.*2003;18:101-11.
35. Cicero A, Derosa G, Miconi A, et al. Possible role of ubiquinone in the treatment of massive hypertriglyceremia resistant to PUFA and fibrates. *Biomed Pharmacother* 2005 Jul;59:312-7.

(Some content Adapted from SpectraCell Laboratories, Inc.)

Estrogen

Estrogen, the primary female sex hormone, exists in three forms—estrone (E1), estradiol (E2), and estriol (E3). It manages the development and regulation of the female reproduction system and secondary sexual characteristics. Several B vitamins are involved in the production of estrogen. Consequently, deficiencies can cause problems. A folate deficiency reduces estrogen levels. Additionally, folate detoxifies excess estrogen via the methylation pathway. It also regulates estrogen's effect on genes.[1,2,3] Vitamin B6 protects genes from estrogen-induced damage, thus lowering the risk of hormone related cancers. B6 detoxifies excess estrogen via the methylation pathway. Unfortunately, estrogen-based oral contraceptives cause B6 deficiency.[4,5,6,7]

Other vitamins are also involved in the production of estrogen. Vitamin D regulates the synthesis of estradiol and estrone. It enhances estrogen's protective effect on bones. [8,9,10] Vitamin C increases the most potent form of estrogen (estradiol) in women on hormone therapy. It lowers aromatase (an enzyme that converts testosterone to estrogen) in the ovaries.[11,12,13] Vitamin K inhibits estrogen activity by binding to estrogen receptors. It lowers the ratio of estradiol (a strong estrogen) to estrone (a weaker estrogen).[14,15] Vitamin E deficiency impairs the estrogen detoxification pathway. Some forms of Vitamin E inhibit estrogen action, especially in breast tissue. Low levels are linked to higher estrogen.[1,16,17] Vitamin A helps to metabolize the biologically active estrogen (estradiol) to an inactive form (estriol).[18,19]

Minerals are critical to the production and control of estrogen. Calcium-D-glucarate lowers estradiol levels. It helps to breakdown estrogen in the liver and convert it to a less toxic form.[1,20,21] Estrogen levels affect how selenium is distributed to various tissues in the body.[22,23] Magnesium is a cofactor for the enzyme that removes toxic forms of estrogen (catechol-ethyltransferase), and estrogen alters magnesium levels throughout the menstrual cycle.[1,24,25,26] While estrogen lowers the risk of zinc deficiency, zinc is dependent upon proteins that metabolize estrogen.[26,27,28] Finally, the amino acid cysteine prevents oxidation of estrogen into a dangerous form that causes breast cancer.[9,30,31]

Reference List

1. Hall D. Nutritional influences on estrogen metabolism. *Appl Nutr Sci Rep* 2001;1-8

2. Ericson U, Borgquist S., Ivarsson M, et al. Plasma Folate Concentrations Are Positively Associated with Risk of Estrogen Receptor {beta} Negative Breast Cancer in a Swedish Nested Case Control Study. *J Nutr* 2010; 140:1661-1668.

3. Wallock-Montellius L, Villanueva J, Chapin R, et al. Chronic ethanol perturbs testicular folate metabolism and ciency reduces sex hormone levels in the Yucatan micropig. *Biol Reprod* 2007;76;455-465

4. Allgood V, Cidlowski J. Vitamin B6 modulates transcriptional activation by multiple members of the steroid hormone receptor superfamily. *J Biol Chem* 1192;25:3819-3824

5. Zhu B. Medical hypothesis: hyperhomocysteinemia is a risk factor for estrogen-induced hormonal cancer. *Int J Oncol* 2003;22:499-508

6. Tully D, Allgood V, Cidlowski J. Modulation of steroid receptor-mediated gene expression by vitamin B6. *FASEB J* 1994;8:343-349

7. El Sahwy S, Osman M, el-Tabakh S, et al. Effect of the administration of vitamin B6 at two levels of intake on xathurenic acid excretion among oral contraceptive pill users. *J Egypt Public Health Assoc* 1988;63:393-405

8. Somjen D. Vitamin D modulation of the activity of estrogenic compounds in bone cells in vitro and in vivo. *Crit Rev Eukaryot Gene Expr* 2007;17:115-147

9. Parikh G, Varadinova M, Suwandhi P et al. Vitamin D regulates steroidogenesis and insulin-like growth factor binding protein-1 (IGFBP-1) production in human ovarian cells. *Horm Metab Res* 2010;42:754-757.

10. Villaggio B, Soldano S, Cutolo M. 1,25-dihydroxyvitamin D3 downregulates aromatase expression and ammatory cytokines in human macrophages. *Clin Exp Rheumatol* 2012;30:934-938.

11. Vihtamaki T, Parantainen J, Koivisto M, et al. Oral ascorbic acie increases plasma oestrdiol during postmenopausal

hormone replacement therapy. *Maturitas* 2002;25:129-135.

12. Wu X, Iguchi T, Itoh N, et al. Ascorbic acid transported by sodium-dependent vitamin C transporter 2 stimulates steroidogenesis in human choriocarcinoma cells. Endocrinology 2008;149:73-83.

13. Tsuji M, Ito Y, Terado N, et al. Ovarian aromatase activity in scorbutic mutant rats unable to synthesize ascorbic acid. *Acta Endocrinol* 1989;121:595-602.

14. Otsuka M, Kato N, Ichimura T et al. Vitamin K2 binds 17beta-hydorxysteroid dehydrogenase 4 and modulates estrogen metabolism. *Life Sci* 2005;76:2473-2482.

15. Jung J, Ishida K, Nishihara T, et al.Anti estrogenic activity of fifty chemicals evaluated by in vitro assays. *Life Sci* 2004;74:3065-3074

16. Lee H, Ju J, Paul S, et al. Mixed tocopherols prevent mammary tumorigenesis by inhibiting estrogen action and activating PPAR-gamma. *Cancer Res* 2009;15:4242-4249

17. Hshieh T, Wu J. Suppression of cell proliferation and gene expression by combinatorial synergy of EGCG, resveratrol and gamma-tocotrienol in estrogen receptor-positive MCF-7 breast cancer cells. *Int J Oncol*

18. Cheng Y, Yin P, Xue, et al. Retinoic acid (RA) regulates 17beta-hydroxysteroid dehydrogenase type 2 city protein (SP) 1/SP3 for estradiol metabolism. *J Clin Endocrinol Metab* 2008;93:1915-1923.

19. Zhu S, Li Y, Li H, et al. Retinoic acid (RA) regulates 17beta-hydroxysteroid dehydrogenase type 2 city protein (SP) 1/SP3 for estradiol metabolism. *J Clin Endocrinol Metab* 2008;93:1915-1923.

20. Monograph: Calcium-D-Glucarate as a chemopreventive agent in breast cancer. *Isr J Med Sci* 1995;31:101-105.

21. Heerdt A, Young C, Borgen P. Calcium glucarate as a chemopreventive agent in breast cancer. *Isr J Med Sci* 1995;31:101-115.

22. Zhou X, Smith A, Failla M, et al. Estrogen status alters tissue distribution and metabolism of selenium in female rats. *J Nutr Biochem* 2012;23:532-538.

23. Ha E, Smith A. Selenium-dependent glutathione peroxidase activity is increased in healthy postmenopausal women. Biol Trace Elem Res 2009;131:90-95.

---

24. Muneyvirci-Delale O, Nacharaju V, Altura B. Sex steroid hormones modulate serum ionized magnesium and calcium levels throughout the menstrual cycle in women. *Fertil Steril* 1198;69:958-962.
25. Butterworth M, Lau S, Monks T. 17 beta-Estradiol metabolism by hamster hepatic microsomes. Implications for the catechol-O-methyl transderase-mediated detoxication of catechol estrogens. *Drugs Metab Dispos* 1996;24:588-594.
26. Bureau I, Anderson R, Arnaud J, et al. Trace mineral status in post menopausal women: impact of hormonal replacement therapy. *J Trace Elem Med Biol* 2002;16:9-13.
27. Herzberg M, Lusky A, Blonder J. The effect of estrogen replacement therapy on Zinc in serum and urine. *Obstet Gynecol* 1996;87:1035-1040.
28. Favier A. The role of zinc in reproduction. Hormonal mechanisms. *Biol Trace Elem Res* 1992;32:363-382.
29. Cavalieri E, Rogan E. Unbalanced metabolism of endogenous estrogens in the etiology and prevention of human cancer. *J Steroid Biochem Mol Biol* 2011;125:169-180.
30. Venugopal D, Zahid M, Mailander P, et al. Reduction of estrogen-induced transformation of mouse mammary epithelial cells by N-acetylcystein. *J Steroid Biochem Mol Biol* 2008;109:22-30.
31. Zahid M, Saeed M, Ali M, et al. N-acetylcysteine blocks formation of cancer-initiating estrogen-DNA adducts in cells. *Free Radic Biol Med* 2010;49:392-400.
32. Fische rL, da Costa K, Kwoch L. dietary choline requirements of women: effects of estrogen and genetic variation. *Am J Clin Nutr* 2010;92:1113-1119.
33. Corbin k, Zeisal S. The nutrigenetics and nutrigenomics of the dietary requirement for Choline. *Prog Mol Biol Transl Sci* 2012;108:159-177.

Additional references at http://www.spectracell.com/online-library-mnt-adhd-abstracts/
(Some content Adapted from SpectraCell Laboratories, Inc.)

Fatigue

Fatigue may be temporary or chronic. Vitamins are key to preventing it. The B Vitamin biotin helps the liver utilize glycogen for energy. Additionally, animal studies confirm that a biotin deficiency causes clinical fatigue.[1] Vitamin C aids iron uptake and transport. It is a precursor to carnitine and several hormones that affect energy levels. Supplementation reduced fatigue in various studies.[2-4] When cellular levels of Vitamin A are low, mitochondrial respiration and ATP (adenosine tryphosphate—energy currency of life) production decreases.[5] An inverse correlation exists between fatigue and Vitamin E levels.[6] Low levels of Vitamin D are seen in patients with chronic fatigue syndrome. A Vitamin D deficiency also causes reduced muscle strength.[7,8] B Vitamins are necessary for converting food into energy. B Vitamins, including B1, B2, B3, B5, B6, B12 and folate, are cofactors in the mitochondrial respiratory chain.[9,2,10-15]

There are several minerals that may fight fatigue. Magnesium is required to store the energy molecule ATP. Repletion of magnesium in chronic fatigue patients shows clinical improvement in energy levels.[2,10,11] Chromium promotes glucose uptake into cells, helping to stabilize blood sugar.[10,16] A zinc deficiency lowers immunity and may cause muscle fatigue. Zinc is also involved in several biochemical reactions for energy metabolism[2,17,18]

Certain amino acids are important. Asparagine supplementation delayed fatigue during exercise by decreasing the rate at which glycogen was used up. It is needed for gluconeogenesis, a process that allows glucose to be made from protein to prevent blood sugar from getting too low.[19-21] Mental and physical fatigue coincides with reduced levels of the amino acid glutamine in various tissues. Supplementation makes muscle tissue more sensitive to insulin, increasing energy levels.[22-24] Serine thwarts the overproduction of fatigue-causing stress hormones like cortisol.[25,26]

A CoQ10 deficiency causes fatigue due to its role in mitochondrial energy metabolism. Therapeutic benefits have been observed, particularly in chronic fatigue syndrome.[2,27-29] Fructose intolerance, fatigue, and hypoglycemia are classic symptoms of this condition since sugars deplete ATP, the main form of cellular energy.[30,31] Several studies confirm that oxidative stress exacerbates clinical symptoms of fatigue. Mitochondrial dysfunction (inefficient energy metabolism) can be treated therapeutically with antioxidants, such as selenium, cysteine, alpha lipoic acid, and glutathione. Chronic fatigue patients have unusually low levels of these anitoxidants.[29, 30-33] Carnitine transports fatty acids into mitochondria and decreases both mental and physical fatigue in clinical studies.[2, 34,35]

Reference List

1. Osada K, Komai M, et al. Experimental study of fatigue provoked by biotin deficiency in mice. *Int J Vitam Nutr Res* 2004;74:334-340.
2. Werbach M. Nutritional strategies for treating chronic fatigue syndrome. *Altern Med Rev* 2000;5:93-108.
3. Huskisson E, Maggini S, Ruf M. The role of vitamins and minerals in energy metabolism and well-being. *J Int Med Res* 2007;35:277-289.
4. Suh S, Bae W, et al. Intravenous vitamin C administration reduces fatigue in office workers: a double-blind randomized controlled trial. *Nutr J* 2012;11:7.
5. Acin-Perez R, Hoyos B, et al. Control of oxidative phosphorylation by Vitamin A illuminates a fundamental role in mitochondrial energy homeostasis. *FASEB J* 2010; 24: 627-634.
6. Vecchiet J, Cipollone F, et al. relationship between musculoskeletal symptoms and blood markers of oxidative stress in patients with chronic fatigue syndrome. *Neurosci Lett* 2003; 335: 151-154.
7. Berkovitzz S, Ambler G, et al. Serum 25-hydroxyl Vitamin D Levels in Chronic Fatigue Syndrome: A Retrospective Survey. *Int J Vitamin Nutr Res* 2009; 79: 250-254.
8. Shinchuk L, Holick M. Vitamin D and rehabilitation: improving functional outcomes.*Nutr Clin Pract* 2007;22:297-304.
9. Head K, Kelly G. Nutrients and botanicals for treatment of stress: adrenal fatigue, neurotransmitter imbalance, anxiety, and restless sleep. *Altern Med Rev* 2009;14:114-140.
10. Huskisson E, Maggini S, Ruf M. The role of vitamins and minerals in energy metabolism and well-being. *J Int Med Res*

2007;35:277-289.

11. Heap L, Peters T, Wessely S. Vitamin B status in patients with chronic fatigue syndrome. *J R Soc Med* 1999;92:183-185.

12. Shimizu T, Hoshino H, et al. Anti-fatigue effect of dicethiamine hydrochloride is likely associated with excellent absorbability and high transformability in tissues as a Vitamin B(1). *Eur J Pharmacol* 2010;635:117-123.

13. Nozaki S, Mizuma H, et al. Thiamine tetrahydrofurfuryl disulfide improves energy metabolism and physical performance during physical-fatigue loading in rats. *Nutr Res* 2009;29:867-872.

14. Engels A, Schroer U, Schremmer D. Efficacy of a combination therapy with vitamins B6, B12 and folic acid for general feeling of ill-health. Results of a non-interventional post-marketing surveillance study. *MMW Fortschr Med* 2008;149 Suppl 4:162-166.

15. Lundell K, Qazi S, et al. Clinical activity of folinic acid in patients with chronic fatigue syndrome. *Arzeimittelforschung* 2006;56:399-404.

16. Cefalu W, Rood J, et al. Characterization of the metabolic and physiologic response to chromium supplementation in subjects with type 2 diabetes mellitus. *Metabolism* 2010;59:755-762.

17. Maes M, Mihaylova I, et al. In chronic fatigue syndrome, the decreased levels of omega-3 poly-unsaturated fatty acids are related to lowered serum zinc and defects in T cell activation. *Neuro Endocrinol Lett* 2005;26:745-751.

18. Cordova A, Alvarez-Mon M. Behaviour of zinc in physical exercise: a special reference to immunity and fatigue. *Neurosci Biobehav Rev* 1995;19:439-445.

19. Marquezi M, Roschel H, et al. Effect of aspartate and asparagine supplementation on fatigue determinants in intense exercise. *Int J Sport Nutr Exer Metab* 2003;13:65-75.

20. Lancha A, Recco M, et al. Effect of aspartate, asparagine, and carnitine supplementation in the diet on metabolism of skeletal muscle during a moderate exercise. *Physiol Behav* 1995;57:367-371.

21. Efthivoulou M, Phillips J, Berry M. Abolition of the inhibitory effect of ethanol oxidation on gluconeogenesis

from lactate by asparagine or low concentrations of ammonia. *Biochim Biophys Acta* 1995;1244:303-310.

22. Jin G, Kataoka Y, et al. Changes in plasma and tissue amino acid levels in an animal model of complex fatigue. *Nutrition* 2009;25:597-607.

23. Prada P, Hirabara S, et al. L-glutamine supplementation induces insulin resistance in adipose tissue and improves insulin signalling in liver and muscle of rats with diet-induced obesity. *Diabetologia* 2007;50:1949-1959.

24. Greenfield J, Farooqi I, et al. Oral glutamine increases circulating glucagon-like peptide 1, glucagon, and insulin concentrations in lean, obese, and type II diabetic subjects. *Am J Clin Nutr* 2009; 89:109-113.

25. Head K, Kelly G. Nutrients and botanicals for treatment of stress: adrenal fatigue, neurotransmitter imbalance, anxiety, and restless sleep. *Altern Med Rev* 2009;14:114-140.

26. Starks M, Starks S, et al. The effects of phosphatidylserine on endocrine response to moderate intensity exercise. *J Int Soc Sports Nutr* 2008;5:11.

27. Mizuno K, Tanaka M, et al. Antifatigue effects of coenzyme Q10 during physical fatigue. *Nutrition* 2008;24:293- 299.

28. Maes M, Mihaylova I, et al. Coenzyme Q10 deficiency in myalgic encephalomyelitis / chronic fatigue syndrome (ME/CFS) is related to fatigue, autonomic and neurocognitive symptoms and is another risk factor explaining the early mortality in ME/CFS due to cardi. *Neuro Endocrinol Lett* 2009;30:47-476.

29. Logan A, Wong C. Chronic fatigue syndrome: oxidative stress and dietary modifications. *Altern Med Rev* 2001;6:450-459.

30. Guery M, Douillard C, et al. Doctor, my son is so tired... about a case of hereditary fructose intolerance. *Ann Endocrinol* 2007;68:456-459.

31. Litherland G, Hajduch E, et al. Fructose transport and metabolism in adipose tissue of Zucker rats: diminished GLUT5 activity during obesity and insulin resistance. *Mol Cell Biochem* 2004;261:23-33.

32. Maes M, Mihaylova I, et al. Not in the mind of neurasthenic lazybones but in the cell nucleus: patients with chronic

fatigue syndrome have increased production of nuclear factor kappa beta. *Neuro Endocrinol Lett* 2007;28:456-462.

33. Bounous G, Molson J. Competition for glutathione precursors between the immune system and the skeletal muscle: pathogenesis of chronic fatigue syndrome. *Med Hypotheses* 1999;53:347-349.

34. Nicolson G, Conklin K. Reversing mitochondrial dysfunction, fatigue and the adverse effects of chemotherapy of metastatic disease by molecular replacement therapy. *Clin Exp Metastasis* 2008;25:161-169.

35. Malaguarnera M, Cammalleri L, et al. L-Carnitine treatment reduces severity of physical and mental fatigue and increases cognitive functions in centenarians: a randomized and controlled clinical trial. *Am J Clin Nutr* 2007;86:1738-1744.

36. Vermeulen R, Scholte H. Exploratory open label, randomized study of acetyl- and propionylcarnitine in chronic fatigue syndrome. *Psychosom Med* 2004;66:276-282.

(Some content Adapted from SpectraCell Laboratories, Inc.)

Female Fertility

At least 12% of the U.S. female population, age fifteen to forty-four, experiences some infertility.[1] Female fertility is dependent on adequate levels of vitamins. Folate protects genes during rapid cell division, which increases the likelihood of a healthy embryo (via methylation of DNA). A folate deficiency raises homocysteine, which damages reproductive cells.[2-5] Vitamins B6 and B12 are both needed to convert toxic homocysteine to a benign form. Low homocysteine levels are linked to a better chance of pregnancy.[6-9] Vitamin C increases serum progesterone levels. It induces ovulation in some women and also enhances effect of the fertility drug clomiphene.[10-13] Higher levels of Vitamin D are linked to better success rates of IVF (in vitro fertilization). It influences production of the sex hormones estradiol and progesterone.[14-16] Vitamin E protects reproductive cells (follicles). It may improve endometrial response (ability of fertilized egg to implant into uterine wall properly) during IVF.[17-20]

A deficiency of the trace mineral selenium has been implicated in miscarriage and infertility. In one trial, 100% of infertile women achieved pregnancy after supplementation.[21,22] Also, minerals are essential to enzyme processes. The trace elements zinc, copper, and magnesium determining several enzymes, such as superoxide dismutase, are needed to protect a woman's reproductive organs.[23-26]

Certain amino acids are necessary to female fertility. Glutathione protects eggs (fertilized or not) from damage by reactive oxygen species. The protective action of the follicle stimulating hormone on embryonic development is due largely to glutathione synthesis.[23, 27,28] N-acetyl cysteine can boost ovulation and pregnancy rates in women with infertility due to PCOS (polycystic ovary syndrome) when these women have not responded to fertility drugs. It also improves viability of endometrial cells in vitro and is a precursor to glutathione.[29-31] Reproductive cells, including embryos, are very susceptible to damage from oxidative stress due to the rapid rate of growth. A low status of antioxidants can cause infertility or miscarriage.[20,23,32,33] Consequently, taking antioxidants should be considered for fertility problems.

Reference List

1. Centers for Disease Control and Prevention. Infertility. *National Center for Health Statistics.* http://www.cdc.gov/nchs/fastats/infertility.htm. 2016. Accessed 13 Sep 2016.
2. Laanpere M, Altmäe S, Stavreus-Evers A, et al. Folate-mediated one-carbon metabolism and its effect on female fertility and pregnancy viability. *Nutr Rev* 2010;68:99-113.
3. Forges T, Monnier-Barbarino P, Alberto J, et al. Impact of folate and homocysteine metabolism on human reproductive health. *Hum Reprod Update* 2007;13:225-238.
4. Ebisch I, Thomas C, Peters W, et al. The importance of folate, zinc and antioxidants in the pathogenesis and prevention of subfertility. *Hum Reprod Update* 2007;13:163-174.
5. Dawson D, Sawers A. Infertility and folate deficiency. Case Reports. *Br J Obstet Gynaecol* 1982;89:678-680.
6. Ocal P, Ersoylu B, Cepni I, et al. The association between homocysteine in the follicular fluid with embryo quality and pregnancy rate in assisted reproductive techniques. *J Assist Reprod Genet* 2012;29:299-304.
7. Berker B, Kaya C, Aytac R, et al. Homocysteine concentrations in follicular fluid are associated with poor oocyte and embryo qualities in polycystic ovary syndrome patients undergoing assisted reproduction. *Hum Reprod* 2009;24:2293-2302.
8. Ebisch I, Peters W, Thomas C, et al. Homocysteine, glutathione and related thiols affect fertility parameters in the (sub) fertile couple. *Hum Reprod* 2006;21:1725-1733.
9. Jerzak M, Putowski L, Baranowski W. Homocysteine level in ovarian follicular fluid or serum as a predictor of successful fertilization. *Gynekol Pol* 2003;74:949-952.
10. Henmi H, Endo T, Kitajima Y, et al. Effects of ascorbic acid supplementation on serum progesterone levels in patients with a luteal phase defect. *Fertil Steril* 2003;80:459-461.
11. Tannetta D, Sargent I, Linton E, et al. Vitamins C and E Inhibit Apoptosis of Cultured Human Term Placenta Trophoblast. *Placenta* 2008;29:680-690.

---

12. Luck M, Jeyaseelan I, Scholes R. Ascorbic acid and fertility. *Biol Reprod* 1995;52:262-266.
13. Igarashi M. Augmentative effect of ascorbic acid upon induction of human ovulation in clomiphene-ineffective in ovulatory women. *Int J Fertility* 1977;22:168-173.
14. Lerchbaum E, Obermayer-Pietsch B. Vitamin D and fertility: a systematic review. *Eur J Endocrinol* 2012;166:765-778.
15. Anagnostis P, Karras S, Goulis D. Vitamin D in human reproduction: a narrative review. *Int J Clin Pract* 2013;Epub ahead of print.
16. Ozkan S, Jindal S, Greenseid K, et al. Replete vitamin D stores predict reproductive success following in vitro fertilization. *Fertil Steril* 2010;94:1314-1319.
17. Cicek N, Eryilmaz O, Sarikaya E, et al. Vitamin E effect on controlled ovarian stimulation of unexplained infertile women. *J Assist Reprod Genet* 2012;29:325-328
18. Nugent D, Newton H, Gallivan L, et al. Protective effect of vitamin E on ischaemia-reperfusion injury in ovarian grafts. *J Reprod Fertil* 1998;114:341-346.
19. Campos C, Ferriani R, Dos Reis R, et al. Lipid peroxidation and vitamin E in serum and follicular fluid of infertile women with peritoneal endometriosis submitted to controlled ovarian hyperstimulation: a pilot study. *Fertil Steril* 2008;90:2080-2085.
20. Tarin J, Ten J, Vendrell F, et al. Effects of maternal ageing and dietary antioxidant supplementation on ovulation, fertilization and embryo development in vitro in the mouse. *Reprod Nutr Dev*1998;38:499-508.
21. Mistry H, Broughton Pipkin F, Redman C, et al. Selenium in reproductive health. *Am J Obstet Gynecol* 2012;206:21-30.
22. Howard J, Davies S, Hunnisett A. Red cell magnesium and glutathione peroxidase in infertile women – effects of oral supplementation with magnesium and selenium. *Magnes Res* 1994;7:49-57.
23. Fujii J, Iuchi Y, Okada F. Fundamental roles of reactive oxygen species and protective mechanisms in the female reproductive system. *Reprod Biol Endocrinol* 2005;3:43.
24. Pathak P, Kapil U. Role of trace elements zinc, copper and magnesium during pregnancy and its outcomes. *Indian J Pediatr* 2004;71:1003-1005.

25. Noda Y, Ota K, Shirasawa T, et al. Copper/zinc superoxide dismutase insufficiency impairs progesterone secretion and fertility in female mice. *Biol Reprod* 2012;86:1-8.
26. Cetin I, et al. Role of micronutrients in the periconceptual period. *Hum Reprod Update* 2010;16:80-95.
27. Tsai-Turton M, Luderer U. Opposing effects of glutathione depletion and follicle-stimulating hormone on reactive oxygen species and apoptosis in cultured preovulatory rat follicles. *Endocrinology* 2006;147:1224-1236.
28. Gardiner C, Salmen J, Brandt C. Glutathione is present in reproductive tract secretions and improves development of mouse embryos after chemically induced glutathione depletion. *Biol Reprod* 1998;59:431-436.
29. Badawy A, State O, Abdelgawad S. N-acetyl cysteine and clomiphene citrate for induction of ovulation in polycystic ovary syndrome: a cross-over trial. *Acta Obstet Gynecol Scand* 2007;86:218-222.
30. Rizk A, Bedaiwy M, Al-Inany H. N-acetyl cysteine is a novel adjuvant to clomiphene citrate in clomiphene citrate-resistance patients with polycystic ovary syndrome. *Fertil Steril* 2005;83:367-270.
31. Estany s, Palacio J, Barnadas R, et al. Antioxidant activity of N-acetylcysteine, flavonoids and alpha-tocopherol on endometrial cells in culture. *J Reprod Immunol* 2007;75:1-10.
32. Agarwal A, Gupta S, Sharma R. Role of oxidative stress in female reproduction. *Reprod Biol Endocrinol* 2005;3:28.
33. Ruder E, Hartman T, Blumberf J, et al. Oxidative stress and antioxidants: exposure and impact on female fertility. *Hum Reprod Update* 2008;14:345-357.

(Some content Adapted from SpectraCell Laboratories, Inc.)

Fibromyalgia

Fibromyalgia, a chronic disorder, is characterized by widespread musculoskeletal pain, fatigue, and tenderness in localized areas. It affects about 2% of the population. Choline and inositol are involved in pain perception, and their levels are altered in fibromyalgia.[1-4] Because low Vitamin D levels impair neuromuscular function and cause muscle pain, a Vitamin D deficiency is common in fibromyalgia patients.[5-9] Additionally, a Vitamin B1 (thiamin) deficiency mimics fibromyalgia symptoms, which are serotonin depletion (decreased pain threshold), a decrease in repair enzymes (muscle soreness), and poor energy production (muscle fatigue).[10,11]

Mineral supplements are important in the treatment of fibromyalgia. Low zinc blood levels are associated with a number of tender points in fibromyalgic patients, and zinc supplements have relieved pain for some.[12] Also, magnesium is involved in pain perception pathways and muscles contraction. Treatment with magnesium can improve tenderness and pain.[13-15] Selenium deficiency has been linked to fibromyalgia. In one trial, symptoms improved in 95% of patients receiving supplements of selenium for at least four weeks.[15-17]

As with many other conditions, antioxidants and certain amino acids relieve the symptoms. Fibromyalgia is often considered an oxidative stress disorder. A low antioxidant status contributes to the pain. Clinical studies consistently show that CoQ10 reduces fibromyalgia symptoms, such as pain and fatigue.[18-21] Low antioxidant status increases pain in fibromyalgia, which is often considered an oxidative stress disorder.[22-24] A carnitine deficiency causes muscle pain due to inefficient cellular energy metabolism (mitochondrial myopathy) that exhibits as fibromyalgia.[25,26] The blood levels of the amino serine are much lower in fibromyalgia patients, indicating a need for supplementation.[27,28]

Reference List

1. Fayed N, Garcia-Campayo J, Magallón R, et al. Localized 1H-NMR spectroscopy in patients with fibromyalgia: a controlled study of changes in cerebral glutamate/glutamine,

inositol, choline, and N-acetylaspartate. *Arthritis Res Ther* 2010;12:R134.
2. Wang S, Su D, Wang R, et al. Antinociceptive effects of choline against acute and inflammatory pain. *Neuroscience* 2005;132:49-56.
3. Petrou M, Harris R, Foerster B, et al. Proton MR Spectroscopy in the Evaluation of Cerebral Metabolism in Patients With Fibromyalgia: Comparison With Healthy Controls and Correlation With Symptom Severity. *Am J Neuroradiol* 2008;29:913-918.
4. Galeotti N, Bartolini A, Gherlardine C. Role of intracellular calcium in acute thermal pain perception. *Neuropharmacology* 2004;47:935-944.
5. Turner M, Hooten W, Schmidt J, et al. Prevalence and Clinical Correlates of Vitamin D Inadequacy among Patients with Chronic Pain. *Pain Med* 2008;9:979-984.
6. Shinchuk L, Holick M. Vitamin D and rehabilitation: improving functional outcomes. *Nutr Clin Pract* 2007;22:297-304.
7. Al-Allaf A, Mole P, Paterson C, et al. Bone health in patients with fibromyalgia*Rheumatology* 2003;42:1202-1206.
8. Plotnikoff F, Quigley J. Prevalence of severe hypovitaminosis D in patients with persistent, nonspecific musculoskeletal pain. *Mayo Clin Proc* 2003;78:1463-1470.
9. Mascarenthas R, Mobarhan S. Hypovitaminosis D-induced pain.*Nutr Rev* 2004;62:354-9.
10. Eisinger J. Alcohol, thiamin and fibromyalgia. *J Am Coll Nutr* 1998;17:300-302.
11. Koike H, Watanabe H, Inukai A, et al. Myopathy in thiamine deficiency: analysis of a case. *J Neurol Sci* 2006;249:175-179.
12. Sendur OF, Tastaban E, Turan Y, et al. The relationship between serum trace element levels and clinical parameters in patients with fibromyalgia. *Rheumatol Int* 2008;28:1117-1121.
13. Magaldi M, Moltoni L, et al. Changes in intracellular calcium and magnesium ions inthe physiopathology of the fibromyalgia syndrome. *Minerva Med* 2000;91:137-140.
14. Abraham G, Flechas J. Management of fibromyalgia: rationale for the use of magnesium and malic acid. *J Nutr*

Ab *Med* 1991;3:49-59.
15. Eisinger J, Plantamura A, Marie P, et al. Selenium and magnesium status in fibromyalgia. *Magnes Res* 1994;7:285-288.
16. Chariot P, Bignani O. Skeletal muscle disorders associated with selenium deficiency in humans. *Muscle Nerve* 2003;27:662-668.
17. Reinhard P, Schweinsberg F, Wernet D, et al. Selenium status in fibromyalgia. *Toxicol Lett* 1998;96-97:177-180.
18. Cordero M, Alcocer-Gomez E, de Miguel M, et al. Coenzyme Q(10): A novel therapeutic approach for Fibromyalgia? Case series with 5 patients. *Mitochondrion* 2011;11:623-625.
19. Lister R. An open, pilot study to evaluate the potential benefits of coenzyme Q10 combined with Ginkgo biloba extract in fibromyalgia syndrome. *J Int Med Res* 2002;30:195-199.
20. Cordero M, Moreno-Fernandez A, Demiguel M, et al. Coenzyme Q10 distribution in blood is altered in patients with Fibromyalgia. *Clin Biochem* 2009;42:732-735.
21. Altindag O, Celik H. Total antioxidant capacity and the severity of the pain in patients with fibromyalgia. *Redox Rep* 2006;11:131-135.
22. Ozgocmen S, Ozyurt H, et al. Antioxidant status, lipid peroxidation and nitric oxide in fibromyalgia: etiologic and therapeutic concerns. *Rheumatol Int* 2006;26:598-603.
23. Bagis S, Tamer L, Sahin G, et al. Free radicals and antioxidants in primary fibromyalgia: an oxidative stress disorder? *Rheumatol Int* 2005;25:188-190.
24. Abdullah M, Vishwanath S, Elbalkhi A, et al. Mitochondrial myopathy presenting as fibromyalgia: a case report. *J Med Case Rep* 2012;6:55.
25. Rossini M, di Munno O, Valentini G, et al. Double-blind, multicenter trial comparing acetyl l-carnitine with placebo in the treatment of fibromyalgia patients. *Clin Exp Rheumatol* 2007;25:182-188.
26. Yunus M, Dailey J, Aldag J, et al. Plasma tryptophan and other amino acids in primary fibromyalgia: a controlled study. *J Rheumatol* 1992;19;90-94.
27. Koning T, Klomp L. Serine-deficiency syndromes. *Curr*

Opin Neurol 2004;17:197-204.

(Some content Adapted from SpectraCell Laboratories, Inc.)

Gastrointestinal (GI) Health

Recent studies confirm the importance of good gastrointestinal health to the overall health of the body. Some common gastrointestinal disorders include chronic constipation, diverticulitis, gastroesophageal reflux disease, inflammatory bowel diseases, irritable bowel syndrome, and ulcers. Vitamins, minerals, amino acids, and antioxidants are needed to maintain GI health.

Vitamin A regulates growth of epithelial cells, including those that line the gastrointestinal (GI) tract, and reduces inflammatory proteins in the gut.[1,2] An inflamed gut uses up the antioxidant Vitamin C faster than a healthy gut. Vitamin C promotes tissue healing in the GI tract and also reduces gastrointestinal inflammation.[3,4] Vitamin D keeps the gut flora healthy by protecting good bacteria. It activates adaptive immunity that originates in the GI tract and promotes gut barrier integrity. A Vitamin D deficiency co-occurs with inflammatory bowel disease flare-ups.[5-7] Vitamin K is synthesized by the bacteria in the intestines. Consequently, a deficiency is common in chronic GI disorders. A deficiency of Vitamin K co-occurs with inflammatory bowel diseases, such as Crohn's and ulcerative colitis.[8,9]

B Vitamins are essential for good health. Vitamin B12 improves gastrointestinal complaints in some patients who have dyspepsia (indigestion). In fact, antacids diminish B12.[10,11] Vitamin B6 deficiency co-occurs with a higher risk of developing colon cancer.[12,13] A folate deficiency alters genes in a way that makes colon cells more likely to become cancerous.[14,15] Choline sustains the barrier function of gastric epithelium (helps prevent stomach ulcers) via its role in building cell membranes and acting as a surfactant in the GI tract, which acts a deterrent to bacteria, specifically yeast entering the body.[16,17]

There are several minerals that aid digestion in the GI tract. Selenium is a cofactor to glutathione peroxidase (GPx0), which protects the intestinal wall from inflammatory damage. Lower GPx activity due to a selenium deficiency is very common in people with gut inflammation.[18-20] Zinc decreases intestinal permeability. It maintains the integrity of the intestinal wall, especially when inflammatory chemicals (TNFa) compromise epithelial lining. It works with Vitamin A in regenerating cells that line the gut.[21-23] Magnesium deficiency affects the amount of good bacteria found in the gut and may help prevent stomach ulcers. Insufficient levels are very common in people with irritable bowel syndrome. Antacids actually induce magnesium deficiency.[24-26]

Amino acids are essential. Glutathione counteracts oxidative stress in the intestinal mucosa (gut wall). It recycles antioxidants, such as Vitamins C and E.[27-29] Glutamine is the preferred fuel for enterocytes (small intestine cells), which use the most glutamine in the entire body. It keeps the junctions between the intestinal epithelial cells tight so foreign proteins cannot enter the bloodstream.[30-32] Carnitine may be useful therapeutically in people with colitis (inflammation of colon) due to its role in fatty acid metabolism, which is often impaired in GI disorders.[33-35] Finally, lipoic acid reduces damaging chemicals (cytokines) in the GI tract that cause an inflammatory immune response and preserves glutathione levels and recycles Vitamin C.[36,37]

Reference List

1. Long K, Santos J, et al. Vitamin A supplementation reduces the monocyte chemoattractant protein-1 intestinal immune response of Mexican children. *J Nutr* 2006;136:2600-2605.
2. Bai A, Lu N, Guo Y, et al. All-trans retinoic acid down-regulates inflammatory responses by shifting the Treg/Th17 profile in human ulcerative and murine colitis. *J Leukoc Biol.* 2009;86:959–969.
3. Aghkassi E, Wendland B, Steinhart H, et al. Antioxidant vitamin supplementation in Crohn's disease decreases oxidative stress: a randomized controlled trial. *Am J Gastroenterol* 2003;98:348-353.
4. Cevikel MH, Tuncyurek P, Ceylan F, et al. Supplementation with high-dose ascorbic acid improves intestinal anastomotic healing. *Eur Surg Res.* 2008;40:29-33.
5. Palmer M, Weaver C. Linking vitamin D deficiency to inflammatory bowel disease. *Inflamm Bowel Dis* 2013;19:2245-2256.
6. Ulitsky A, Ananthakrishnan AN, Naik A, et al. Vitamin D deficiency in patients with inflammatory bowel disease: association with disease activity and quality of life. *J Parenter Enteral Nutr.* 2011 May;35:308-316.
7. Blanack S. Vitamin D deficiency is associated with

ulcerative colitis disease activity. *Dig Dis Sci.*2013;58:1698-1702.

8. Nakajima S, Iijima H, Egawa S, et al. Association of vitamin K deficiency with bone metabolism and clinical disease activity in inflammatory bowel disease. *Nutrition.* 2011 Oct;27:1023-1028.

9. Schoon E, Muller M Vermeer C, et al. Low serum and bone vitamin K status in patients with longstanding Crohn's disease: another pathogenic factor of osteoporosis in Crohn's disease? *Gut* 2001;48:473-477.

10. Gumurdulu Y, Serin E, Ozer B, et al. The impact of B12 treatment on gastric emptying time in patients with Helicobacter pylori infections. *J Clin Gastroenterol* 2003;37:230-233.

11. Oh S. Proton pump inhibitors – uncommon adverse effects. *Aust Fam Physician* 2011;40:705-708.

12. Larsson S, Orsini N, Wolk A. Vitamin B6 and Risk of Colorectal Cancer: A Meta-analysis of Prospective Studies. *JAMA* 2010;303:1077-1083.

13. Lee J, Li H, Giocannucci E, et al. Prospective study of plasma vitamin B6 and risk of colorectal cancer in men. *Cancer Epidemiol Biomarkers Prev* 2009;18:1197-1202.

14. Crott J, Liu Z, et al. Moderate folate depletion modulates the expression of selected genes involved in cell cycle, intracellular signaling and folate uptake in human colonic epithelial cell lines.*J Nutr Biochem* 2008;19:328-335.

15. Knock E, Deng L, Wu Q, et al. Low dietary folate initiates intestinal tumors in mice, with altered expression of G2-M checkpoint regulators polo-like kinase 1 and cell division cycle 25c. *Cancer Res* 2006;66:10359-10356.

16. Mourelle M, Guarner F, Malagelada J. Polyunsaturated phosphatidylcholine prevents stricture formation in a rat model of colitis. *Gastroenterolgy* 1996;110:1093-1097.

17. Dunjic B, Axelson J. Gastroprotective capability of exogenous phosphatidylcholine in experimentally induced chronic gastric ulcers in rats. *Scand J Gastroenterol* 1993;28:89-94.

18. Esworthy R, Binder S, Doroshow J, et al. Microflora trigger colitis in mice deficient in selenium-dependent glutathione

peroxidase and induce Gpx2 gene expression. *Biol Chem.* 2003;384:597-607.

19. Nagy D, Fülesdi B, Hallay J. Role of selenium in gastrointestinal inflammatory diseases. *Orv Hetil* 2013;154:1636-1640.

20. Brigelius-Flohé R, Kipp A. Physiological functions of GPx2 and its role in inflammation-triggered carcinogenesis. *Ann N Y Acad Sci.* 2012;1259:19-25.

21. Ranaldi G, Ferruzza S, Canali R, et al. Intracellular zinc is required for intestinal cell survival signals triggered by the inflammatory cytokine TNFα. *J Nutr Biochem* 2013;24:967-976.

22. El Tawil A. Zinc supplementation tightens leaky gut in Crohn's disease. *Inflamm Bowel Dis* 2012;18:E399.

23. Zhong W, McClain C, Cave M, et al. The role of zinc deficiency in alchohol-induced intestinal barrier dysfunction. *Am J Physiol Gastrointest Liver Physiol* 2010;298:G625-633.

24. Pachikian BD, Neyrinck AM, Deldicque L, et al. Changes in intestinal bifidobacteria levels are associated with the inflammatory response in magnesium-deficient mice. *J Nutr.* 2010;140:509-514.

25. Mackay J, Bladon P. Hypomagnesaemia due to proton-pump inhibitor therapy: a clinical case series.*QJM.* 2010;103:387-395.

26. Henrotte J, Aymard N, Allix M, et al. Effect of pyridoxine and magnesium on stress-induced gastric ulcers in mice selected for low or high blood magnesium levels. *Ann Nutr Metab* 1995;39:285-290.

27. Sido B, Hack V, Hochlehnert A, et al. Impairment of intestinal glutathione synthesis in patients with inflammatory bowel disease. *Gut.* 1998;42:485-492.

28. Pinto M, Soares-Mota S, Lopes M, et al. Does active Crohn's disease have decreased intestinal antioxidant capacity? *J Crohns Colitis* 2013;7:e358-e366.

29. Esworthy R, Binder S, Doroshow J, et al. Microflora trigger colitis in mice deficient in selenium-dependent glutathione peroxidase and induce Gpx2 gene expression. *Biol Chem.* 2003;384:597-607.

30. Li N, Neu J. Glutamine deprivation alters intestinal tight junctions via a PI3K/Akt mediated pathwas in Caco-2 cells.

J Nutr 2009;139:710-714.

31. Lecleire S, Hassan A, Marion-Letellier R. et al. Combined glutamine and arginine decrease proinflammatory cytokine production by biopsies from Crohn's patients in association with changes in nuclear factor-kappaB and p38 mitogen-activated protein kinase pathways. *J Nutr* 2008;138:2481-2486.

32. Li J, Langkamp-Henken B, Suzuki K, et al Glutamine prevents parenteral nutrition-induced increases in intestinal permeability. *J Parent Enteral Nutr* 1994;18:303-307.

33. Sonne S, Shekhawat PS, Matern D, et al. Carnitine deficiency in OCTN2-/- newborn mice leads to a severe gut and immune phenotype with widespread atrophy, apoptosis and a pro-inflammatory response. *PLoS One.* 2012;7:e47729.

34. Mikhailova T,Sishkova E, Poniewierka E, et al. Randomised clinical trial: the efficacy and safety of propionyl-L-carnitine therapy in patients with ulcerative colitis receiving stable oral treatment. *Aliment Pharmacol* 2011;34:1088-1097.

35. Shekhawat P, Srinivas S, Matern D, et al. Spontaneous development of intestinal and colonic atrophy and inflammation in the carnitine-deficient jvs (OCTN2(-/-)) mice. *Mol Genet Meta.* 2007;92:315-324.

36. Trivedi P, Jena G. Role of α-lipoic acid in dextran sulfate sodium-induced ulcerative colitis in mice: Studies on inflammation, oxidative stress, DNA damage and fibrosis. *Food Chem Toxicol.* 2013;59:339-55.

37. Kolgazi M, Jahovic N, Yüksel M, et al. Alpha-lipoic acid modulates gut inflammation induced by trinitrobenzene sulfonic acid in rats. *J Gastroenterol Hepatol.* 2007;22:1859-1865.

(Some content Adapted from SpectraCell Laboratories, Inc.)

Headaches

Headaches are one of the most common disorders of the nervous system and can be associated with a variety of other disorders. Some vitamins can help to prevent headaches. Foremost are a number of B Vitamins. Vitamin B3, niacin, dilates blood vessels and increases serotonin.[1,2] Vitamin B9, folate, scavenges nitric oxide, which is implicated in migraine pathogenesis.[3,4] Vitamin B2, riboflavin, is effective for migraine prevention as it aids mitochondrial energy metabolism.[5,6] The MTHFR gene has been linked to migraines, and this gene raises folate requirements.[7-8] Vitamin C has a newly discovered role in neural tissue, which may explain its clinical benefit in a double-blind trial on headache frequency.[9,10] Several small trials show effectiveness in a combination treatment of Vitamin D and calcium.[11,12]

In addition to calcium, other minerals are necessary. Magnesium is the most important mineral, especially in regards to migraines. It has been efficacious in several migraine trials. A magnesium deficiency can create arterial spasm, and its role in neurotransmission may explain the migraine-magnesium depletion co-occurence.[13-16] The antioxidant CoQ10 aids mitochondrial metabolism, so it may prevent migraines.[17-21] Two amino acids are related to migraines. Carnitine is implicated in migraine pathophysiology due to its role in mitochondrial energy metabolism from fatty acids.[22] Low levels of glutathione peroxidase have been implicated in migraine etiology.[24] Finally, lipoic acid enhances mitochondrial energy metabolism.[23]

Reference List

1. Prousky J, Seely D. The treatment of migraines and tension-type headaches with intravenous and oral niacin (nicotinic acid): systematic review of the literature. *Nutr J* 2005;4:3.
2. Velling DA, Dodick DW, Muir JJ. Sustained-release niacin for prevention of migraine headache. *Mayo Clin Proc* 2003;78:770-771.
3. Di Rosa G, Attina S, et al. Efficacy of folic acid in children with migraine, hyperhomocysteinemia and MTHFR polymorphisms. *Headache* 2007;47:1342-1344.
4. Van der Kuy P, Merkus F. et al. Hydroxocobalamin, a nitric

oxide scavenger, in the prophylaxis of migraine: an open, pilot study. *Cephalalgia* 2002;22:513-519.

5. Boehnke C, Reuter U, et al. High-dose riboflavin treatment is efficacious inmigraine prophylaxis: an open study in a tertiary care centre. *Eur J Neurol* 2004;11:475-477.

6. Breen C, Crowe A, et al. High dose riboflavin for prophylaxis of migraine. *Can Fam Physician* 2003;49:1291-1293.

7. Lea R, Colson N. The effects of vitamin supplementation and MTHFR (C677T) genotype on homocysteine-lowering and migraine disability. *Pharmacogenet Genomics* 2009;19:422-428.

8. Schurks M, Rist PM, et al. MTHFR 677C>T and ACE D/I polymorphisms in migraine: a systematic review and meta-analysis. *Headache* 2010:50:588-599.

9. Bali L, Callaway E. Vitamin C and migraine: a case report. *N Engl J Med* 1978;299:364.

10. Calero CI, Vickers E, et al. Allosteric Modulation of Retinal GABA Receptors by Ascorbic Acid. *J Neurosci* 2011;31:9672-9682.

11. Thys-Jacob S. Alleviation of migraines with therapeutic vitamin D and calcium. *Headache* 1994;34:590-592.

12. Prakash S, Shah ND. Chronic tension-type headache with vitamin D deficiency: casual or causal association? *Headache* 2009;49:1214-1222.

13. Grazzi L, Andrasik F, et al. Magnesium as a treatment for paediatric tensiontype headache: a clinical replication series. *Neurol Sci* 2005;25:338-341.

14. Grazzi L, Andrasik F, et al. Magnesium as a preventive treatment for paediatric episodic tension-type headache: results at 1-year follow-up. *Neurol Sci* 2007;28:148-150.

15. Durlach J, Pages N, et al. Headache due to photosensitive magnesium depletion. *Magnes Res* 2005;18:109-122.

16. Wang F, Van Den Eeden SK, et al. Oral magnesium oxide prophylaxis of frequent migrainous headache in children: a randomized, double-blind, placebo-controlled trial. *Headache* 2003;43:601-610.

17. Slater SK, Nelson TD, et al. A randomized, double-blinded, placebo controlled, crossover, add-on study of CoEnzyme

Q10 in the prevention of pediatric and adolescent migraine. *Cephalalgia* 2011;31:897-905.

18. Hershey AD, Powers SW, et al. Coenzyme Q10 deficiency and response to supplementation in pediatric and adolescent migraine. *Headache* 2007;47:73-80.
19. Sandor PS, Afra J. Nonpharmacologic treatment of migraine. *Curr Pain Headache Rep* 2005;9:202-205.
20. Sandor PS, Di Clemente L, et al. Efficacy of coenzyme Q10 in migraine prophylaxis: a randomized controlled trial. *Neurology* 2005;64:713-715.
21. Bianchi A, Salomone S, et al. Role of magnesium, coenzyme Q10, riboflavin, and vitamin B12 in migraine prophylaxis. *Vitam Horm* 2004;69:297-312.
22. Kabbouche MA, Powers SW, et al. Carnitine palmityltransferase II (CPT2) deficiency and migraine headache: two case reports. *Headache* 2003;43:490-495.
23. Magis D, Ambrosini A, et al. A randomized double-blind placebo-controlled trial of thioctic acid in migraine prophylaxis. *Headache* 200747:52-57.
24. Bolayir E, Celik K, et al. Intraerythrocyte antioxidant enzyme activities in migraine and tension-type headaches. *J Chin Med Assoc* 2004;67:263-267.

(Some content Adapted from SpectraCell Laboratories, Inc.)

Heart Disease

Since 1900, heart disease has been the number one killer of Americans and is the leading cause of death worldwide. One in three Americans currently has some form of heart disease. Over 150,000 deaths with people under the age of sixty-five from heart disease occur each year in the U.S. Cardiovascular disease ranks as the number two cause of death, after accidents, for children under fifteen years of age. Several factors, including blood pressure (see Hypertension section), arterial scarring, and build up of plague, contribute to heart disease.

Several vitamins prevent arterial scarring, a cause of heart attacks. Vitamin B6, B12, folate, and choline together are necessary to properly metabolize homocysteine and reduce the risk of arterial scarring.[1,2] Vitamin B1 (thiamine) is another vital component in energy metabolism by helping the heart increase its pumping strength. Deficiencies of Vitamin B1 have been found in patients with congestive heart failure and in the long-term use of diuretic drugs, which are often prescribed to those patients and deplete the body's storage of thiamine.[3,4] Vitamin B3 (niacin) lowers blood cholesterol (fats in the blood), inhibits the oxidation of LDL, and is currently the most effective drug available for raising the heart-protective, good HDL cholesterol.[5,6] One study on side products made from Vitamin B5 (pantothenic acid) demonstrated a decrease in blood triglycerides and cholesterol.[7] Another study showed that inositol, a member of the B Vitamin family, decreases dangerous small, dense lipoproteins that easily penetrate blood vessel walls and cause artherosclerosis.[8] B-vitamin therapy has been an effective treatment for reducing heart disease and blood pressure, high blood pressure being associated with heart attacks.[9,10]

There are several micronutrients that influence blood pressure, which can result in physical damage to the walls of the blood vessels. Vitamin D deficiency is linked to hypertension because it contributes to endothelial dysfunction, a condition in which the lining of blood vessels cannot relax properly and secretes substances that promote inflammation of the blood vessel lining.[11,12] Although the causes of hypertension often overlap, micronutrient deficiencies can create or worsen this condition. Vitamin K and Vitamin A with absorption facilitated by oleic acid reduce the build up of plague in the arteries.[13,14] Additional evidence suggests that

Vitamin E can even retard existing atherosclerosis.[15]

Several mineral deficiencies, such as zinc, copper, calcium and magnesium, co-occur with high blood pressure.[17-19] Deficiencies in minerals—calcium, magnesium, zinc, and selenium—contribute to the symptoms of congestive heart failure.[20] Additionally, drinking "hard" water that contains naturally occurring magnesium, calcium, copper, and zinc correlates with a lower risk of heart attacks.[21] As to be expected, certain amino acids are necessary. Carnitine, an amino acid, facilitates the transport of fatty acids into heart cell mitochondria, thus helping the heart to meets its strong demand for chemical energy. It also helps muscles, including the heart, to recover from damage, such as from a heart attack.[20,21]

Studies also indicate that a high level of oxidative stress eventually takes its toll on arteries, ultimately causing hypertension. Several studies of coenzyme Q10 showed that it lowered blood pressure significantly. Is also required by cardiac tissue in large amounts to properly function.[22, 23] The antioxidant Vitamins C and E help blood vessels maintain their flexibility, allowing them to easily dilate and contract. The powerful antioxidant lipoic acid decreases blood pressure by impeding inflammatory responses in the blood vessels.[24,25]

Scientists now emphasize that heart disease is in reality an inflammatory condition within the blood vessels. Inflammation and oxidative stress work together to damage arteries, impairing cardiac function. Several antioxidant nutrients diminish this inflammatory process. Glutathione, an amino acid, is the most potent intracellular antioxidant and actually helps to regenerate other antioxidants in the body. Cysteine, glutathione, B2, selenium, Vitamin E, and Vitamin C cooperate to reduce oxidative stress throughout the complete cardiovascular system.[27,28]

Reference List

1. Olszewski AJ, Szostak WB, Bialkow M, Rudnicki S. Reduction of plasma lipid and homocysteine levels by pyridoxine, folate, cobalamin, choline, riboflavin, and troxerutin in atherosclerosis. *Atherosclerosis* Volume 75, Issue 1, January 1989, pages 1-6.
2. Spence JD. Homocysteine-lowering therapy: a role in stroke prevention? *The Lancet Neurology* Volume 6, Issue 9,

September 2007, Pages 830–838.
3. Shimon H, Almog S, Vered Z, et al. Improved left ventricular function after thiamine supplementation in patients with congestive heart failure receiving long-term furosemide therapy. *The American Journal of Medicine* Volume 98, Issue 5, May 1995, Pages 485-490.
4. Seligmann H, Halkin H, Rauchfleisch S. Thiamine deficiency in patients with congestive heart failure receiving long-term furosemide therapy: a pilot study. *The American Journal of Medicine* Volume 91, Issue 2, August 1991, Pages 151-155.
5. The AIM-HIGH Investigators. The role of niacin in raising high-density lipoprotein cholesterol to reduce cardiovascular events in patients with atherosclerotic cardiovascular disease and optimally treated low-density lipoprotein cholesterol: Rationale and study design. The Atherothrombosis Intervention in Metabolic syndrome with low HDL/high triglycerides: Impact on Global Health outcomes (AIM-HIGH). *American Heart Journal* Volume 161, Issue 3, March 2011, Pages 471–477.e2.
6. Taylor AJ, Sullenberger LE, Lee HJ, Lee JK, Grace KA. Arterial Biology for the Investigation of the Treatment effects of Reducing Cholesterol (ARBITER)2 A Double-Blind, Placebo-Controlled Study of Extended-Release Niacin on Atherosclerosis Progession in Secondary Prevention Patients treated With Statins. *Circulation*, 2004;110:3512-3517.
7. McCarty MF. Inhibition of acetyl-CoA carboxylase by cystamine may mediate the hypotriglyceridemic activity of pantethine. *Medical Hypotheses* Volume 56, Issue 3, March 2001, Pages 314-317.
8. Grases FJ, Prieto RM, Simonet BM, Torres JJ. Dietary *myo*-inositol hexaphosphate prevents dystrophic calcifications in soft tissues: a pilot study in Wistar rats. *Life Sciences* Volume 75, Issue 1, 21 May 2004, Pages 11–19.
9. The Heart Outcomes Prevention Evaluation (HOPE) 2 Investigators* Homocysteine Lowering with Folic Acid and B Vitamins in Vascular Disease. *N Engl J Med* 2006; 354:1567-1577April 13, *2006*DOI: 10.1056/NEJMoa060900

---

10. van Guildener C, Prabath WB, Nanayakkara C, Stehouwer DA. Homocystein and blood pressure. *Current Hypertension Reports* January 2003, 5:26.
11. Stricker H, Bianda FT, Guidicelli-Nicolosi S, Limoni C, Colucci G. Effect of a Single, Oral, High-dose Vitamin D Supplementation on Endothelial Function in Patients with Peripheral Arterial Disease: A Randomised Controlled Pilot Study. *European Journal of Vascular and Endovascular Surgery* Volume 44, Issue 3, September 2012, Pages 307–312.
12. Mheid IA, Patel R, Murrow J, Morris A. Vitamin D status is associated with arterial stiffness and vascular dysfunction in healthy humans.. *J Am Coll Cardio* Volume 58, Issue 2, July, 2001.
13. Kon-Siong GJ, Bots ML, Vermeer C, Witteman JCM, Grobbee DE. Vitamin K intake and osteocalcin levels in women with and without aortic atherosclerosis: a population-based study. *Atherosclerosis* Volume 116, Issue 1, July 1995, Pages 117-123.
14. Visioli F, Bellomo G, Montedoro GF, Galli C. Low density lipoprotein oxidation is inhibited in vitro by olive oil constituents. *Atherosclerosis* Volume 117, Issue 1, September 1995, Pages 25-32.
15. Salonen RM, Nyyssonen K, Kaikkonene J. Six-Year Effect of Combined Vitamin C and E Supplementation on Atherosclerotic Progression. The Antioxidant Supplementation in Atherosclerosis Prevention (ASAP) Study. *Circulation* 2003;107:947-953.
16. Houston MC. Nutraceuticals, vitamins, antioxidants, and minerals in the prevention and treatment of hypertension. *Progress in Cardiovascular Diseases,* May-June, 20015, Volume 47, Issue 6, Pages 396-449.
17. Houston MC. Treatment of hypertension with nutraceuticals, vitamins, antioxidants and minerals. Expert Review of Cardiovascular Therapy, Volume , 2007, Issue 4.
18. Alsafwah A, LaGuardia S, Arroyo, M, et.al. Congestive Heart Failure is a Systemic Illness: A Role for Minerals and Micronutrients. *Clin Med Res* 2007 Dec; 5(4) PMC2275753.
19. Frost FJ. *Studies of minerals and cardiac health in selected populations.*

---

http://www.who.int/water_sanitation_health/dwq/nutrientsch ap8.pdf. Accessed 17 Sep 2016.

20. Lango R, Smolenski RT. Influence of L-carnitine and its derivatives on myocardial metabolism and function in ischemic heart disease and during cardiopulmonary bypass. *Cardiovascular ...*, 2001 - cardiovascres.oxfordjournals.org.

21. Arsenian MA. Carnitine and its derivatives in cardiovascular disease. *Progress in Cardiovascular Diseases* Volume 40, Issue 3, November–December 1997, Pages 265-286.

22. Rosenfeldt FL, Haas SJ, Krum H, et al. Coenzyme Q_{10} in the treatment of hypertension: a meta-analysis of the clinical trials. *Journal of Human Hypertension* (2007) 21, 297–306.

23. Burke BE, Neuenschwander R, Olson RD. Randomized, Double-Blind, Placebo-Controlled Trial of Coenzyme Q10 in Isolated Systolic Hypertension. *Southern Medical Journal* Nov. 2001;1112+.

24. Ting HH, Timimi FK, Haley EA, Roddy MA, Ganz P. Vitamin C improves endothelium-dependent vasodilation in forearm resistance vessels of humans with hypercholesterolemia. *Circulation* 1997;95:2617-2622.

25. Nunes GL, Robinson K, Kalynych A, King SB. Viatmins C and E inhibit O2-production in the pig coronary artery. *Circulation* 1997;96:3593-3601.

26. Midaoui AEL, Elimadi A, Wu L. Lipoic acid prevents hypertension, hyperglycemia, and the increase in heart mitochondrial superoxide production. *American J of Hypertension*:16(3):173-179.

27. Aviram M. Review of human studies on oxidative damage and antioxidant protection related to cardiovascular diseases. *Free Radical Research* [2000, 33 Suppl:S85-97].

28. Halliwell B, Zentella A, Gomez EO. Antioxidants and human disease: a general introduction. *Nutrition,* Nutrition Reviews.55.1. (Jan 1997): S44-9; discussion S49-52.

Some content adapted from SpectraCell Laboratories, Inc.

Hypertension

Hypertension, high blood pressure, is associated with heart disease and is also discussed in that section. There are several vitamins that work to prevent hypertension. In pharmacological doses, biotin, a B Vitamin, reduced systolic blood pressure by activating an enzyme (cGMP) that causes smooth muscles to relax.[1,2] People with a certain gene called MTHFR type TT tend to respond well to B2 therapy for lowering blood pressure.[3,4] Vitamin B6 decreases homocysteine, a toxin that makes arteries stiff and raises blood pressure. Low B6 co-occurs with hypertension. [5-8] Folate reduces blood pressure by improving endothelial function, or the ability of blood vessels to properly dilate.[9,10]

Vitamin A restrains the growth of vascular smooth muscle, thus keeping blood vessels (lumen) clear and wide.[11,12] Vitamin C improves the ability of blood vessels to react appropriately to relaxation signals, and it increases nitric oxide, a powerful vasodilator. [13-15] Low Vitamin D is strongly linked to hypertension, possibly due to its role in calcium transport. It augments blood pressure lowering the effect of calcium. It also keeps the blood vessels smooth and healthy [13,16, 17] Vitamin E increases nitric oxide synthase, an enzyme that causes blood vessels to dilate. It protects blood vessels from damage.[18,19]

Certain minerals also affect hypertension. Optimal calcium status reduces vasoconstriction. Calcium is particularly effective for salt sensitive hypertension as it increases sodium excretion.[13,20,21] Magnesium encourages dilation of blood vessels. Low intracellular levels of magnesium are a known cause of hypertension.[22-24] Copper regulates enzymes that keep blood vessels dilating properly. Its depletion causes hypertension. Supplementation trials have been positive.[25-28] Zinc manages angiotensin and endothelin, two enzymes that directly affect blood pressure. A zinc deficiency causes blood vessels to constrict.[29]

Antioxidants help with hypertension. Coenzyme Q10 improves the bioenergetics of the blood vessel wall. A deficiency positively correlates to hypertension. However, benefits of CoQ10 are often not seen for several weeks.[13, 30,31] Lipoic acid improves the vascular tone and causes vasolidation. It works like calcium channel blocker medications and also recycles Vitamins C and E and cysteine. [32]

Amino acids that help to prevent hypertension include cysteine, carnitine, and glutathione. Cysteine's anti-hypertensive effects stem from its role as a potent antioxidant. It is an effective vasolidator.[33,34] Carnitine lowers blood pressure in the same way as ACE inhibitors, a common hypertension drug that reduces angiotensin, a substance that causes arteries to constrict. Its role in fat metabolism explains this effect.[35,36] Oxidative stress, which often manifests as glutathione deficiency, can induce hypertension.[37]

Finally, oleic acid found in olive oil and nuts benefits blood pressure. Oleic acid protects endothelial cells (inner lining of blood vessels) from inflammation.[38]

Reference List

1. Watanabe-Kamiyama M, Kamiyama S, Horiuchi K, et al. Antihypertensive effect of biotin in stroke-prone spontaneously hypertensive rats. *Br J Nutr* 2008;99:656-763.
2. Rodriguez-Melendez R, Zempleni J. Nitic oxide signaling depends upon biotinin Jurkat human lymphoma cells. *J Nutr* 2009;139:429-433.
3. Horigan G, McNully H, Ward M, et al. riboflavin lowers blood pressure in cardiovascular disease patients from homozygous for the 677C-T polymorphism in MTHFR. *J Hypertens* 2010;28:478-486.
4. Wilson C, McNully H, Scott J, et al. Postgraduate Synposium: The MTHFR C677T polymorphisms, B-vitamins and blood pressure. *Proc Nutr Sci* 2010;69:156-165.
5. Preston I, Tang G, Tilan J, et al. Retenoids and pulmonary hypertension. *Circulation* 2005; 111:782-790.
6. Neuville P, Bochaton-Piallat M, Gabbianni G. retenoids and arterial smooth muscle cells. *Arterioscler Thromb Vasc Biol* 200;20:1882-1888.
7. Stehouwer C, vanGuldener C. Does homocysteine cause hypertension? *Clin Chem Lab Med* 2003;41:408-411.
8. Lin P, Cheng C, Wei J, et al. Low plasma pyridoxal 5'-phosphate concentration and MtHFR 677C-T genotypes are associated with increased risk of hypertension. *Int J Vitamin Nutr Res* 2008;78:33-43.
9. McRae M. High-dose folic acid supplementation effects on

endothelial function and reduces blood pressure in hypertensive patients: a meta-analysis of randomized controlled clinical trials. *J Chiropr Med* 2009;8:15-24.

10. Mongoni A, Sherwood R, Swift C, et al. Folic acid enhances endothelial function and reduces blood pressure in smokers: a ramdomized controlled trail. *J Inter Med* 2002;252:407-503.

11. Preston I, Tang G, Tilan J, et al. Retenoids and pulmonary hypertension. *Circulation* 2005; 111:782-790.

12. Neuville P, Bochaton-Piallat M, Gabbianni G. retenoids and arterial smooth muscle cells. *Arterioscler Thromb Vasc Biol* 200;20:1882-1888.

13. Houston M. The role of vascular biology, nutrition, and nutrceuticals in the prevention and treatment of hypertension. *J Am Nutraceutical Assoc* 2002; Supplement No. 1;5:5-71.

14. May J. How does ascorbic acid prevent endothelial dysfunction? *Free Rad Biol Med* 2000;28:1421-1429.

15. Juraschek S, Gualler E, Appel L, et al. Effects of Vitamin C supplementation on blood pressure: ameta-analysis of randomized controlled trials. *Am J Clin Nutr* 2012;95:1079-1088.

16. Hanni L, Huafner L, Sorenson O, et al. Viatmin D is related to blood pressure and other cardiovascular risk factors in middle-aged men. *Am J Hypertens* 1995;8:894-901.

17. MacCarthy E, Yamashita W, Hsu A, et al. 1,25 hydroxy Vitamin D3 and rat vascular smooth muscle cell growth. *Hypertension* 1989;13:954-959.

18. Newaz W, Newal N, Rohaizan C, et al. a- Tocopherol increased nitric oxide synthase activity in blood vessels of spontaneously hypertensive rats. *Am J Hypertens* 1999;12:839-844.

19. Mottram P, Shige H, Nestal P. Vitamin E improves arterial compliance in middle-aged men and women. *Atheroslerosis* 1999;145:399-404.

20. Weinberger M, Wagner U, Fineberg N. The blood pressure effects of calcium supplementation in humans known sodium responsiveness. *Am J Hypertens* 1993;6:799-805.

21. Mc Carron D. Calcium metabolism and hypertension. *Keio J Med* 1995;44:105-114.

22. Barbagallo M, Dominguez L, Resnick L. Magnesium metabolism in hypertension and type 2 diabetes mellitus.

Am J Ther 2007;14:375-385.
23. Jees S, Miller E, Gualler E, et al. The effect of magnesium supplementation on blood pressure: a meta-analysis of randomized clinical trials. *Am J Hypertens* 2002;15:691-696.
24. Touyz R. Role of magnesium in the pathogenesis of hypertension. *Mol Aspects Med* 2003; 60:476-496.
25. Ozumi K, Sudhahar V, Kim H, et al. Role of copper transport proteinantioxidant 1 in angiotensin II-induced hypertension; a key regulator of extrcellular superoxidase dismutase. *Hypertension* 2012; 60:476-486.
26. Kievay L. Endothelial dysfunction, isoprostanes, and copper deficiency. *Hypertension* 2008;52:e27.
27. Alarcon O, Guerrero Y, Ramirez M, et al. Effect of copper supplementation on blood pressure values in patients with stable moderate hypertension. *Arch Latinoam Nutr* 2003; 53:271-276.
28. Rosenfeldt F, Haas s, Krum H, et al. Coenzyme Q10 in the treatment of hypertension: a meta-analysis of the clinical trails. *J Hum Hypertens* 2007;21:296-306.
29. Weissmann N. Nitric-oxide-mediated zinc release: a new (modulatory) pathway in hypoxic pulmonaryvasoconstriction. *Circ Res.* 2008 Jun 20;102(12):1451-4. doi: 10.1161/CIRCRESAHA.108.178962. No abstract available. PMID:18566310.
30. Langsjoen P, Willis R, Galkers K. Treatment of essential hypertension with coenzyme Q10. *Mol Aspects Med* 1994;15:S265-S272.
31. Han W, Zhu D, Wu L, et al. N-acetylcysteine-induced vasodilation involves voltage-gated potassium channel in rat aorta. *Life Sci* 2009;84:732-737.
32. Moura FA, de Andrade KQ, dos Santos JC, Goulart MO. Lipoic Acid: its antioxidant and anti-inflammatory role and clinical applications. *Curr Top Med Chem.* 2015;15(5):458-83. Review. PMID: 25620240.
33. Ruggenenti P, Cattaneo D, Loriga G, et al. Ameliorating hypertension and insulin resistance in sbjects at increased risk: effects of aceyl-L-carnitine therapy. *Hypertension* 2009;54:557-574.
34. Miguel-Carrasco JL, Monserrat MT, Mate A, et al.

Comparative effects of captopril and L-carnitine on blood pressure and antioxidant enzyme gene expression in the heart of spontaneously hypertensive rats. *Eur J Pharmacol* 2010;632:65-72.

35. Ferrar L, Raimondi A, D'Episcopo L, et al. Olive oil and reduced need for hypertensive medications. *A Inter Med* 2000;160:837-842.

36. Ruiz-Gutierrez V, Muriana F, Guerro A, et al. Plasma lipids, ertythrocyte membrane lipids and bllod pressure of hypertensive women after ingestion of dietary oleic acid from two different sources. *J Hypertens* 1996;14:1483-1490.

37. Oelze M, Kröller-Schön S, Steven S, et al. Glutathione peroxidase-1 deficiency potentiates dysregulatory modifications of endothelial nitric oxide synthase and vascular dysfunction in aging. *Hypertension.* 2014 Feb;63(2):390-6. doi: 10.1161/HYPERTENSIONAHA.113.01602. Epub 2013 Dec 2. PMID: 24296279.

38. Harvey K, Walker C, Xu Z, et al. Oleic acid inhibits stearic acid-induced inhibition of cell growth and pro-inflammatory responses in human aortic endothelial cells. *J Lipid Res* 2010;51:3470-3480.

Some content adapted from SpectraCell Laboratories, Inc.

Hypothyroidism

Women are five to eight times more likely than men to have thyroid problems.[1] The majority of people with hypothyroidism are unaware of this condition. Untreated, this problem can affect overall health adversely. Having adequate intake of vitamins is essential for prevention and correction. Deficiencies of B6, B12, or folate (B9) can cause elevated homocysteine that is linked with hypothyroidism. Folic acid levels have been linked to levels of thyroid stimulating hormone (TSH).[2-5] When liver detoxification has been compromised, Vitamin C and E partially restores thyroid function.[6-10] Vitamin A activates a gene that regulates TSH (thyroid stimulating hormone).[11-13] Hypothyroidism negatively influences choline function in the brain. This condition can affect mood and cognition.[14,15]

Along with vitamins, several minerals also help. A deficiency in zinc increases thyroid hormone T3.[16-20] Low levels of copper, seen in experimentally induced hypothyroidism, indirectly affects thyroid status through its antioxidant role via superoxide dismutase.[17] Selenium converts thyroid hormones T4 (thyroxine) into T3 (triiodothyronine) while a deficiency reduces T3 levels, causing classic hypothyroidism symptoms, such as fatigue, depression, and/or weight gain.[18-22]

Asparagine is the amino acid that is part of the structure of thyroid stimulating hormone that regulates communication with other hormones.[24, 25] Antioxidants are also necessary as hypothyroidism decreases the effectiveness of some antioxidants, such as glutathione peroxidase and superoxide dismutase.[25,26] Reduced levels of carnitine in body tissue in both hypo- and hyperthyroidism contribute to muscle fatigue.[27-29] Lipoic acid increases endothelial function in people whose hypothyroidism is not readily observable. It also protects thyroid cells from oxidative stress, but may interfere with T4 therapy.[30,31]

The most critical nutrient for the production of T4, thyroxine, by the thyroid gland is iodine. Iodine deficiency has been well known, especially in the Goiter Belt of the U.S., for many years. It was this fact that prompted the U.S. government to mandate iodized salt for the American population. Although larger goiters are not as common as they used to be, I see many enlarged thyroid glands in my practice and observe them every day in the general population.

Reference List

1. American Thyroid Association. General information/Press room. http://www.thyroid.org/media-main/about-hypothyroidism/. 2016. Accessed 16 Sep 2016.

2. Ibrahaim W, Tousson E, El-Masry T, et al. The effect of folic acid as an antioxidant on the hypothalamic monoamines in experimentally induced hypothyroid rat. *Toxicol Ind Health* 2011 Epub ahead of print.

3. Lippi G, Montagnana M, Targher G, et al. Prevalence of folic acid and vitamin B12 deficiencies in patients with thyroid disorders. *Am J Med Sci* 2008;336:50-52.

4. Evrengul H, Tanriverdi H, Enli Y et al. Interaction of plasma homocysteine and thyroid hormone concentrations in the pathogenesis of the slow coronary flow phenomenon. *Cardiology* 2007;108:186-192.

5. Stella G, Spada R, Calabrese S, et al. Association of thyroid dysfunction with vitamin B12, folate and plasma homocysteine levels in the elderly: a population-based study in Sicily. *Clin Chem Lab Med* 2007;45:143-147.

6. Kowalczyk E, Urbanowicz J, Kopff M, et al. Elements of oxidation/reduction balance in experimental hypothyroidism. *Endokrynol Pol* 2011;62:220-223.

7. Kelly GS. Peripheral metabolism of thyroid hormones: a review. *Altern Med Rev* 2000;5(4):306-333.

8. Gupta P, Kar A. Role of ascorbic acid in cadmium-induced thyroid dysfunction and lipid peroxidation. *J Appl Toxicol* 1998;18:317-320.

9. Chaurasia S, Kar A. Protective effects of vitamin E against lead-induced deterioration of membrane associated type-I iodothyronine 5'-monodeiodinase (5'D-I) activity in male mice. *Toxicology* 1997;124:203-209.

10. Yu J, Shan Z, Chong W, et al. Vitamin E ameliorates iodine-induced cytotoxicity in thyroid. *J Endocrinol* 2011;209:299-306.

11. Zimmermann M, Jooste P, Mabapa N, et al. Vitamin A supplementation in iodine-deficient African children decreases thyrotropin stimulation of the thyroid and reduces the goiter rate. *Am J Clin Nutr* 2007;86:1040-1044.

12. Zimmermann M. Interactions of vitamin A and iodine

deficiencies: effects on the pituitary-thyroid axis. *Int J Vitam Nutr Res* 2007;77:236-240.

13. Beibinger R, Arnold M, Langhans W, et al. Vitamin A repletion in rats with concurrent vitamin A and iodine deficiency affects pituitary TSHbeta gene expression and reduces thyroid hyperstimulation and thyroid size. *J Nutr* 2007;137:537-577.

14. Sawin S, Brodish P, Carter C, et al. Development of cholinergic neurons in rat brain regions: dose dependent effects of propylthiouracil-induced hypothyroidism. *Neurotoxicol Teratol* 1998;20:627-635.

15. Modi S, Bhattacharya M, Sekhri T, et al. Assessment of the metabolic profile in Type 2 diabetes mellitus and hypothyroidism through proton MR spectroscopy. *Magn Reson Imaging* 2008;26:420-425.

16. Nishiyama S, Futagoishi-Suginohara Y, Matsukura M, et al. Zinc supplementation alters thyroid hormone metabolism in disabled patients with zinc deficiency. *J Am Coll Nutr* 1994;13:62-67.

17. Fujimoto S, Indo Y, Higashi A, et al. Conversion of thyroxine into tri-iodothryonine in zinc deficient rat liver. *J Pediatr Gastroenterol Nutr* 1986;5:799-805.

18. Alturfan A,, Zengin E, Dariyerli N et al. Investigation of zinc and copper levels in methimazoleinduced hypothyroidism: relation with the oxidant-antioxidant status. *Folia Biol* 2007;53:183-188.

19. Moncayo R, Kroiss A, Oberwinkler M, et al. The role of Se, vitamin C, and zinc in benign thyroid diseases and of Se in malignant thyroid diseases: low Se levels are found in subacute and silent thyroiditis and in papillary and follicular carcinoma. *BMC Endocr Disord* 2008;8:2.

20. Kralik A, Eder K, Kirchgessner M. Influence of zinc and selenium deficiency on parameters relating to thyroid hormone metabolism. *Horm Metab Res* 1996;28:223-226.

21. Olivieri O, Girelli D, Stanzial A, et al. Selenium, zinc and thyroid hormones in healthy subjects: low T3/T4 ratio in the elderly is related to impaired selenium status. *Biol Trace Elem Res* 1996;51:31-41.

22. Arthur J, Nicol F, Beckett G, et al. Selenium deficiency, thyroid hormone metabolism, and thyroid hormone

deiodinases. *Am J Clin Nutr* 1993;57:236S-239S.
23. Russo D, Chazenbalk G, Nagayama Y, et al. Site-directed mutagenesis of the human thyrotropin receptor: role of asparagine-linked oligosaccharides in the expression of a functional receptor. *Mol Endocrinol* 1991;5:29-33.
24. Fares F, Gruener N, Kraiem Z. The role of the asparagine-linked oligosaccharides of the alphasubunit in human thyrotropin bioactivity. *Endocrinology* 1996;137:555-560.
25. Faustino L, Pires R, Lima A, et al. Liver glutathione S-transferase expression is decreased by 3,5,3-triiodothyronine in hypothyroid but not in euthyroid mice. *Exp Physiol* 2011;96:790-800.
26. Kowalczyk E, Urbanowicz J, Kopff M, et al. Elements of oxidation/reduction balance in experimental hypothyroidism. *Endokrynol Pol* 2011;62:220-223.
27. Benvenga S. Effects of L-carnitine on thyroid hormone metabolism and on physical exercise tolerance. *Horm Metab Res* 2005;37:566-571.
28. Sinclair C, Gilchrist J, Hennessey J, et al. Muscle carnitine in hypo- and hyperthyroidism. *Muscle Nerve* 2005;32:357-359.
29. Benvenga S, Amato A, Calvani M, et al. Effects of carnitine on thyroid hormone action. *Ann NY Acad Sci* 2004;1033:158-167.
30. Gd X, Jh P, Hi S, Ls Z. Alpha-lipoic Acid Improves Endothelial Dysfunction in Patients with Subclinical Hypothyroidism. *Exp Clin Endocrinol Diabetes* 2010;118:625-629.
31. Segermann J, Hotze A, Ulrich H, et al. Effect of alpha-lipoic acid on the peripheral conversion of thyroxine to triiodothyronine and on serum lipid-, protein- and glucose levels. *Arzneimittelforschung* 1991;41:1294-1298.

Some content adapted from SpectraCell Laboratories, Inc.

Inflammation

There is mounting evidence that inflammation is associated with a variety of diseases, including asthma, chronic peptic ulcer, tuberculosis, rheumatoid arthritis, and many more.[1] Poor nutrition contributes to this condition. Low vitamin C co-occurs with inflammation, which is inversely related to C-reactive protein (CRP), a marker for inflammation. Vitamin C also increases the amino acid glutathione.[2-4] Vitamin D is a potent modulator of inflammation. It helps to turn off chronic inflammatory responses and inhibits pro-inflammatory cytokine production.[5,6] Vitamin E limits destructive cell behavior created by inflammatory enzymes gone wild and decreases damage from tumor necrosis factor alpha (TNF-a). Additionally, a vitamin E deficiency predisposes a person to inflammation-related diseases.[7,8]

B Vitamins are always important. A Vitamin B6 deficiency is linked to high levels of CRP and systemic inflammation.[9,10] Vitamin B2 helps to minimize pain associated with inflammation while it detoxifies homocysteine, an amino acid that indirectly causes inflammation in various tissues.[11,12] Finally, Vitamin A manages the cellular immune response to inflammatory signals. A Vitamin A deficiency increases the severity of chronic inflammation.

Minerals act in conjunction to vitamins to improve this condition. For example, zinc depletion lowers vitamin A status.[13-15] Inflammation raises the demand for zinc. Pro-inflammatory chemicals (cytokines) dose dependently decrease in response to zinc repletion.[16-18] Manganese is a cofactor to the powerful antioxidant superoxide dismutase that fights inflammation within cells.[19,20] A magnesium deficiency activates pro-inflammatory chemicals called cytokines. A manganese deficiency also initiates a damaging immune response by activating cells called leukocytes and macrophages.[21-23] A copper deficiency reduces enzyme activity, such as superoxide dismutase, that fights inflammation and also lowers damaging isoprostanes, a by-product of inflammation.[24-26] A selenium deficiency negatively alters genes that regulate the inflammatory response and promotes vascular inflammation.[27,28]

Some amino acids combat inflammation. Glutathione, for example, repairs damage to cells caused by inflammation. It regulates the production of pro-inflammatory cytokines and also recycles Vitamins C and E.[28,29] Cysteine, a precursor to glutathione production, safeguards organs, such as blood vessels, brain, and liver, from inflammatory damage. Supplementation with N-acetyl cysteine raises glutathione.[30-32] Glutamine, a precursor to glutathione, reduces cytokine production and invokes an anti-inflammatory response.[33,34]

There are two antioxidants that are important to reducing inflammation. Lipoic acid (LA) nullifies free radicals caused by uncontrolled inflammation in both water and lipid phases of the cell. Lipoic acid protects endothelial cells from inflammation and regenerates antioxidants, such as Vitamin E, C and glutathione.[35,36]. Coenzyme Q10 decreases several inflammatory markers (CRP and IL-6) in supplementation trials. It affects genes that control inflammatory response.[37-39]

Reference List

1. Nordquist C. Inflammation: Causes, Symptoms and Treatment. *Medical News Today.* http://www.medicalnewstoday.com/articles/248423.php. 16 Sep 2015. Accessed 16 Sep 2016.
2. Mah E,Mmatos M, Kawiecki D, et al. Vitamin C status is related to proinflammatory response and impaired vascular endothelial function in healthy, college-aged lean and obese men. *J Am Diet Assoc* 2011;111:737-743.
3. Mikirova N, Casciari J, Rogers A, et al. Effect of high dose intravenous vitamin C on inflammation in cancer patients. *J Transl Med* 2012;10:189.
4. Lenton K, Sane A, Therriault H, et al. Vitamin C augments lymphocyte gluatathione in subjects with ascorbate deficiency. *Am J Clin Nutr* 2003;77:189-195.
5. Zhang Y, Leung D, Richers b. Viatmin D inhibits monocyte/macrophage proinflammatory cytokine production by targeting MAPK phosphatase-1. *J Immunol* 2012;88:2127-2135.
6. Quefeld U. Vitamin D and inflammation. *Pediatr Neprtol* 2013;28:605-10.
7. Wells S, Jennins M, Rome C, et al. Alpha-, gamma- and delta-tocopherols reduce inflammatory angiogenesis in human microvascular endothelial cells. *J Nutr Biochem* 2010;21:589-597.

8. Yachi R, Muto C, Ohtaka N, et al. Effects of tocotrienol on tumor necrosis factor-a/d-galctosamine-induced steatohepatitis in rats. *J Clin Biochem Nutr* 2013;52:146-153.

9. Ulvik A, Midttun O, Ringdal E et al. Association of plasma B-6 vitamers with systemic markers of inflammation and after pyridoxine treatment in patients with stable angina pectoris. *Am J Clin Nutr* 2012;95:1072-1078.

10. Morris M, Sakakeeny L, Jacques P, et al. Vitamin B-6 intake is inversely related to, and the requirement is affected by, inflammation status. *J Nutr* 2010;140:103-110.

11. Bertollo C, Oliveira A, Rocha L, et al. Characterization of the antnociceptive and anti-inflammatory activities of riboflavin in different experimental models. *Eur J Pharmacol* 2006;547:184-191.

12. Granados-Soto V, Teran-Rosales F, Rocha-Gonzales H, et al. Riboflavin reduces hyperalgesia and inflammation but not tactile allodynia in the rat. Eur J Pharmacol 2004; 492:35-40.

13. Garcia O. Effect of vitamin deficiency on the immune respose in obesity. *Proc Nutr Soc* 2012;71:290-297.

14. Christian P, West K. Interactions between zinc and vitamin A: an update. *Am J Clin Nutr*1998;68:435S-441S.

15. Kim C. Retinoic acid, immunity, and inflammation. *Vitam Horm* 2011;86:83-101.

16. Foster M, Samman S. Zinc and regulation of inflammatory cytokines: implications for cardiometabolic disease. *Nutrients* 2012;4:676-694.

17. Wessels I, Haase H, Engelhardt G, et al. Zinc deficiency induces production of pro-inflammatory cytokines IL-1B and TNFa in promyeloid cells via epigenetic and redox-dependent mechanisms. *J Nutr Biochem* 2013;24:289-297.

18. Costarelli L, Muti E, Malavolta M, et al. Distinctive modulation of inflammatory and meatbolic parameters in relation to zinc nutritional status in adult overweight/obese subjects. *J Nutr Biochem* 2010;21:432-7.

19. Li C, Zhou H. The role of manganese superoxide dismutase in inflammation disease. *Enzyme Res* 2011;387176

20. Holley A, Dhar S, Xu Y et al. Manganese superoxide dismutase: beyond life and death. *Amino Acids* 2012;42:139-158.

---

21. Wglicki W. Hypomagnesemia and inflammation: clinical and basic aspects. *Annu Rev Nutr* 2012;32:55-71.
22. Sugimoto J, Romani A, Valentin-Torres A, et al. Magnesium decreses inflammatory cytokine production: anovel innate immunomodulatory mechanism. *J Immunol* 2012;188:6338-6346.
23. Mazur A, Majer J, Rock E, et al. Magnesium and the infalmamtory response: potential physiopathological implications. *Arch Boichem Biophys*. 2007;458;48-56.
24. Bo S, Durazzo M, Cambino R, et al. Association of dietary and serum copper with inflammation, oxidative stress, and metabolic variables in adults. *J Nutr* 2008;138:305-10.
25. Schuschke D, Adeagbo A, Patibandla P, et al. Cycloxygenase-2 is upregulated I copper-deficient rats. *Inflammation* 2009;32:333-9.
26. DiSilvestro RA, Selsby J, Siefker K. A pilot study of copper supplementation effects on plasma F2alpha isoprostanes and urinary collagen crosslinks in young adult women. *J Trace Elem Med Biol* 2010l;24:165-168.
27. Kipp A, Banning A, van Schothorst E, et al. Marginal selenium deficiency down-regulates inflammation-related genes in splenic leukocytes of the mouse. *J Nutr Biochem* 2012;23:1170-1177.
28. Cao Y, Reddy C, Sordillo L. Altered eicosanoid biosynthesis in selenium-deficient endothelial cells. *Free Radic Biol Med* 2000:28:381-389.
29. Lubos E, Kelly N, Oldebeken S, et al. Glutathine peroxidase-1 deficeincy augments proinflammatory cytokine-induced redox signaling and human endothelial cell activation. *J Biol Chem* 2011;286:35407-35417.
30. Ramires R, Ji L. Glutathione supplementation and training increases myocardial resistance to ischemia-reperfusion in vivo. *Am J Physiol Heart Circ Physiol* 2001;281:H679-H688.
31. Erickson M, Hansen K, Banks W. Inflammation-induced dysfunction of the low-density liopprtein receptor-related protein -1 at the blood-brain barrier: protection by the antioxidant N-acetylcysteine. *Brain Behav Immun* 2012;26:1085-1094.

32. Sekhar R, Patel S, Guthikonda A, et al. Deficient synthesis of glutathione underlies oxidative stress in aging and can be corrected by dietary cysteine and glycine supplementation. *Am J Clin Nutr* 2011;94:847-853.

33. Kim H. Glutamine is an immunonutrient. *Yonsei Med J* 2011;52:892-897.

34. Garret-Cox R, Stefanutti G, Booth C, et al. Gluatmine decreases inflammation in infant rat endotoxemia. *J Pediatr Surg* 2009;44:523-9.

35. Jones W, Li X, Qu Z et al. Uptake, recycling, and antioxidant actions of alpha-lipoic acid in endothelial cells. *Free Radic Biol Med* 2002;33:83-93.

36. Shay K, Moreau R, Smith E, et al. Alpha-lipoic acid as a dietary supplement: molecular mechanisms and therapeutic potential. *Biochim Biophys Acta* 2009;1790:1149-1160.

37. Lee B, Huang y, Chen S, et al. Effects of coenzyme Q10 in inflammation markers (high-sensitivity C-reactive protein, interleukin-6, and homocysteine) in patients with coronary artery disease. *Nutrition* 2012;28:767-72.

38. Ulvik A, Midttun O, Ringdale, et al. Functions of Coenzyme Q10 in inflammation and gene expression. *Biofactors* 2008;32:179-83.

39. Sohet F, Neyrinck A, Pachikian B et al. Coenzyme Q10 supplementation lowers hepatic oxidative stress and inflammation associated with diet-induced obesity in mice. *Biochem Pharmacol* 2009;78:1391-400.

Some content adapted from SpectraCell Laboratories, Inc.

Insomnia

Insomnia affects about 30% of the adult population worldwide. This includes difficulty falling asleep, difficulty with maintaining sleep, waking up too early, and in some cases not feeling rested after sleep.[1] Research shows that taking supplements can help. In clinical trials with Vitamin B1 (thiamine), supplementation of healthy individuals who had marginal B1 deficiency improved their sleep.[2-4] Vitamin B3 (niacin) increases REM (rapid eye movement) sleep while it improves both quality and quantity of sleep by converting tryptophan to serotonin.[5,6] Folate and Vitamin B6 are cofactors for several neurotransmitters in the brain, such as serotonin and dopamine, that regulate sleep patterns. [5,7-10] Vitamin B12 normalizes circadian rhythms (sleep-wake cycles). Studies verify therapeutic benefits of B12 supplementation in both oral and intravenous forms.[11-14] Studies with Vitamin A suggest that a deficiency alters brains waves in non-REM sleep, causing sleep to be less restorative.[15,16]

Improving magnesium status is associated with better quality sleep because it mimics the action of melatonin. It also alleviates insomnia due to restless leg syndrome.[17-21] Both zinc and copper interact with NMDA (N-methyl-Daspartate) receptors in the brain that regulate sleep. A higher zinc to copper ratio is linked to longer sleep duration.[22,23] Finally, oleic acid, a fatty acid found in olive oil and nuts, is a precursor of oleamide, which regulates the drive for sleep and tends to accumulate in the spinal fluid of sleep-deprived animals. Additionally, oleic acid also facilitates the absorption of Vitamin A.[24-26]

Reference List

1. Roth T. Insomnia: Definition, Prevalence, Etiology, and Consequences. *J Cln Sleep Med* 2007;3: S7-S10.
2. Zadeh S, Begum K. Comparison of nutrient intake by sleep status in selected adults in Mysore, India. *Nutr Res Pract* 2011;5:230-235.
3. Smidt L, Cremin F, Grivetti L, et al. Influence of thiamin supplementation on the health and general well-being of an elderly Irish population with marginal thiamine deficiency. *J Gerontol* 1991;46:M16-M22.
4. WilkinsonT, Hanger H, Elmslie J, et al. The response to

treatment of subclinical thiamine deficiency in the elderly. *Am J Clin Nutr* 1997;66:925-928.

5. Head K, Kelly G. Nutrients and botanicals for treatment of stress: adrenal fatigue, neurotransmitter imbalance, anxiety, and restless sleep. *Altern Med Rev* 2009;14:114-140.
6. Robinson C, Pegram G, Hyde R, et al. The effects of nicotinamide upon sleep in humans. *Biol Psychiatry* 1977;12:139-143.
7. Kelly G. Nutritional and botanical interventions to assist with the adaptation to stress. *Altern Med Rev* 1999;4:249-265.
8. Kelly G. Folates: supplemental forms and therapeutic applications. *Altern Med Rev* 1998;3:208-220.
9. Larzelere M, Wiseman P. Anxiety, Depression, and Insomnia. *Prim Care* 2002;19:339-360.
10. Ebben M, Lequerica A, Spielman A. Effects of pyridoxine on dreaming: a preliminary study. *Percept Mot Skills* 2002;95:135-140.
11. Okawa M, Mishima K, Nanami T et al. Vitamin B12 treatment for sleep-wake rhythm disorders. *Sleep* 1990;13:15-23.
12. Ohta T, Ando K, Iwata T, et al. Treatment of persistent sleep-wake schedule disorders in adolescents with methylcobalamin (vitamin B12). *Sleep* 1991;14:414-418.
13. Chang H, Sei Hm Morita Y, et al. Effects of intravenously administered vitamin B12 on sleep in rat. *Physiol Behav* 1995;57:1019-1024.
14. Ebihara S, Mano N, Kurono N, et al. Vitamin B12 affects non-photic entrainment of circadian locomotor activity rhythms in mice. *Brain Res* 1996;727:31-39.
15. Sei H. Vitamin A and sleep regulation. *J Med Invest* 2008;55:1-8.
16. Kitaaoka K, Hattori A, Chikahisa S, et al. Vitamin A deficiency induces a decrease in EEG delta power during sleep in mice. *Brain Res* 2007;1150:121-130.
17. Durlach J, Pages N, Bac P, et al. Biorhythms and possible central regulation of magnesium status, phototherapy, darkness therapy and chronopathological forms of magnesium depletion. *Magnes Res* 2002;15:49-66.
18. Rondanelli M, Opizzi A, Monteferrario F, et al. The effect of melatonin, magnesium, and zinc on primary insomnia in

long-term care facility residents in Italy: a double-blind, placebo-controlled clinical trial. *J Am Geriatr Soc* 2011;59:82-90.

19. Nielson F, Johnson L, Zeng H. Magnesium supplementation improves indicators of low magnesium status and inflammatory stress in adults older than 51 years with poor quality sleep. *Magnes Res* 2010;23:158-168.

20. Hornyak M, Voderholzer U, Hohagen F, et al. Magnesium therapy for periodic leg movements-related insomnia and restless legs syndrome: an open pilot study. *Sleep* 1998;21:501-505.

21. Popoviciu L, Asgian B, Delast-Popoviciu D, et al. Clinical, EEG, electromyographic and polysomnographic studies in restless legs syndrome caused by magnesium deficiency. *Rom J Neurol Psychiatry* 1993;31:55-61.

22. Song CH, Kim YH, Jung KI. Associations of Zinc and Copper Levels in Serum and Hair with Sleep Duration in Adult Women. *Biol Trace Elem Res* 2012;Epub ahead of print

23. Nevsimalova S, Buskova J, Bruha R, et al. Sleep disorders in Wilson's disease. *Eur J Neurol* 2011;18:184-190.

24. Mueller G, Driscoll W. Biosynthesis of oleamide. *Vitam Horm* 2009;81:55-78.

25. Akanmu M, Adeosun S, Ilesanmi O. Neuropharmalogical effects of oleamide in male and female mice. *Behav Brain Res* 2007;182:88-94.

26. Raju M, Lakshminarayana R, Krishnakantha T, et al. Micellar oleic and eicosapentaenoic acid but not linoleic acid influences the beta-carotene uptake and its cleavage into retinol in rats. *Mol Cell Biochem* 2008;288:7-15.

Some content adapted from SpectraCell Laboratories, Inc.

Male Fertility

Male infertility affects 4.5% to 6% of adult males in North America. It is highest in Africa and Eastern Europe.[1] The addition of micronutrients can address some of the problems. Vitamin A regulates genes that control sperm production (spermatogenesis). A deficiency may lower sperm count.[2-4] Vitamin D increases sperm motility and induces acrosome reaction, a process during which a sperm releases enzymes to allow fusion with an egg. Men with low Vitamin D may have slower sperm.[5,6] Low levels of Vitamin C increase damage to sperm's genetic material. Supplementation improved sperm count, motility, and structure in human trials.[7-9] Vitamin E protects sensitive sperm cell membranes. It enhances sperm's ability to penetrate an egg.[10,11]

Additionally, deficiencies in B Vitamins may also affect male fertility. Vitamin B12 is needed for cellular replication, including spermatogenesis. B12 moves from blood to semen to assist in sperm production, so it may increase sperm count.[12-16] A folate (B9) deficiency may reduce testosterone, which is critical to sperm creation due to its role as a methyl donor in DNA synthesis. The MTHFR (methylenetetrahydrofolate reductase) C677T gene that increases folate requirements is a risk factor for male infertility.[17-19]

Men should also be concerned about mineral intake. Copper and manganese are both cofactors for superoxide dismutase (a very powerful antioxidant) that protects sperm from oxidative damage.[20,21] Selenium is required for sperm maturation, and it protects the lipid shell encasing each sperm (prevents lipid peroxidation), which is especially important since sperm have a very delicate fatty acid composition.[22-24] Zinc supplementation in men with low zinc status is often successful for male infertility. A deficiency lowers testosterone and reduces sperm count.[25-27]

Adequate amino acids and antioxidants are necessary. Glutathione, an amino acid, is a cofactor to the enzyme glutathione peroxidase that assures the structural integrity of sperm. A deficiency compromises sperm motility.[28-30] The amino acid carnitine transports fatty acids, the preferred energy source of sperm, into cells, and significantly improves sperm motility in clinical studies.[31,32]

Sperm are highly susceptible to free radical damage to both their genetic material and cell membrane. Consequently, poor antioxidant status is a documented cause of male infertility.[33,34] Coenzyme Q10 acts as a powerful antioxidant protecting sperm from damage and improves semen bioenergetics through its role in mitochondrial function (helps sperm remain viable). A direct correlation exists between CoQ10 and sperm count and motility.[35,36]

Reference List

1. Argarwal A, Mulgund A, Hamada A, & Chyatte MR. A unique view on male infertility around the globe. *Reprod Biol Endrocrinol,* 2015: 13:37.
2. Hogarth C, Griswold M. The key role of vitamin A in spermatogenesis. *J Clin Invest* 2010;120:956-962.
3. Boucheron-Houston C, Canterel-Thouennon L, Lee T, et al. Long-term vitamin A deficiency induces alteration of adult mouse spermatogenesis and spermatogonial differentiation: direct effect on spermatogonial gene expression and indirect effects via somatic cells. *J Nutr Biochem* 2013;24:1123-1135.
4. Wolgemuth D, Chung S. Retinoid signaling during spermatogenesis as revealed by genetic and metabolic manipulations of retinoic acid receptor alpha. *Soc Reprod Fertil Suppl.*2007;63:11-23.
5. Blomberg, Jensen M, Bjerrum P, Jessen T, et al. Vitamin D is positively associated with sperm motility and increases intracellular calcium in human spermatozoa. *Hum Reprod* 2011 Jun;26:1307-17.
6. Hammoud A, Meikle A, Peterson C, et al. Association of 25-hydroxy-vitamin D levels with semen and hormonal parameters. *Asian J Androl* 2012;14:855-859.
7. Akmal M, Qadri J, Al-Waili N, et al. Improvement in human semen quality after oral supplementation of vitamin C. *J Med Food* 2006;9:440-442.
8. Song G, Norkus E, Lewis V. Relationship between seminal ascorbic acid and sperm DNA integrity in infertile men. *Int J Androl* 2006;29:569-575.
9. Dawson E, Harris W, Rankin W et al. Effect of ascorbic acid on male fertility. *Ann NY Acad Sci* 1987;498:312-323.
10. Chen X, Li Z, Ping P, et al. Efficacy of natural vitamin E on oligospermia and athenospermia: a prospective multi-

centered randomized controlled study of 106 cases. *Natl J of Androl* 2012;18:428-431.

11. Kessopoulou E, Powers H, Sharma K, et al.A double-blind randomized placebo cross-over controlled trial using the antioxidant vitamin E to treat reactive oxygen species associated with male infertility. *Fertil Steril* 1995;64:825-831.

12. Boxmeer J, Smit M, Weber R, et al. Seminal plasma cobalamin significantly correlates with sperm concentration in men undergoing IVF or ICSI procedures. *J Androl* 2007;28:521-527.

13. Kawata T, Tamiki A, Tashiro A, et al. Effect of vitaminB12-deficiency on testicular tissue in rats fed by pair-feeding. *Int J Vitam Nutr Res* 1997;67:17-21.

14. Sandler B, Faragher B. Treatment of oligospermia with vitamin B12. *Infertility* 1984;7:133-138.

15. Murphy L, Mills J, et al. Folate and vitamin B12 in idiopathic male infertility. *Asian J Androl* 2011;13:856-861.

16. Boxmeer J, Smit M, Utomo E, et al. Low folate in seminal plasma is associated with increased sperm DNA damage. *Fertil Steril* 2009;92:548-556.

17. Safarinejad M, Shafiei N, Safarinejad S, et al.Relationship between genetic polymorphisms of methylenetetrahydrofolate reductase (C677T, A1298C, and G1793A) as risk factors for idiopathic male infertility. *Reprod Sci* 2011;18:304-315.

18. Murawski M, Saczko J, Marcinkowska A, et al. Evaluation of superoxide dismutase activity and its impact on semen quality parameters of infertile men. *Folia Histochem Cytobiol* 2007;45 Suppl 1:S123-S126.

19. ShivaM, Gautam A, Verma Y, et al. Association between sperm quality, oxidative stress, and seminal antioxidant activity. *Clin Biochem* 2011;44:319-324.

20. Foresta C, Flohe L, Garolla A, et al. Male fertility is linked to the selenoprotein phospholipid hydroperoxide glutathione peroxidase. *Biol Reprod* 2002;67:967-971.

21. Safarinejad M. Efficacy of selenium and/or N-acetyl-cysteine for improving semen parameters in infertile men: a double-blind, placebo controlled, randomized study. *J Urol* 2009;181:741-51.

22. Scott R, MacPherson A, Yates R, et al. The effect of oral selenium supplementation on human sperm motility. *Br J Urol* 1998;82:76-80.
23. Croxford T, McCormick N, Kelleher S. Moderate zinc deficiency reduces testicular zip6 and zip10 abundance and impairs spermatogenesis in mice. *J Nutr* 2011;141:359-365.
24. Ali H, Baig M, Rana M, et al. Relationship of serum and seminal plasma zinc levels and serum testosterone in oligospermic and azoospermic infertile men. *J Coll Physicians Surg Pak* 2005;15:671-673.
25. Colagar A, Marzonye, Chaichi M. Zinc levels in seminal plasma are associated with sperm quality in fertile and infertile men. *Nutr Res* 2009;29:82-88.
26. Lenzi A, Culasso F, Gandini L, et al. Placebo-controlled, double blind, cross-over trial of glutathione therapy in male infertility. *Hum Reprod* 1993;8:1657-1662
27. Shamsi M,Venkatesh S, Kumar R, et al. Antioxidant levels in blood and seminal plasma and their impact on spermparameters in infertile men. *Indian J Biochem Biophys* 2010;47:38-43.
28. Irvine D. Glutathione as a treatment for male infertility. *Rev Reprod*1996;1:6-12.
29. Zhou X, Liu F, Zhai S. Effect of L-carnitineand/or L-acetyl-carnitine in nutrition treatment for male infertility: a systematic review. *Asia Pac J Clin Nutr* 2007;16 Suppl 1:383-390.
30. Garolla A, Maiorino M, Roverato A, et al. Oral carnitine supplementation increases sperm motility in asthenozoospermic men with normal sperm phospholipid hydroperoxide glutathione peroxidase levels. *Fertil Steril* 2005;83:355-361.
31. Agarwal A, Makker K, Sharma R. Clinical relevance of oxidative stress in male factor infertility: an update. *Am J Reprod Immunol* 2008;59:2-11.
32. Ross C, Morriss A, Khairy M, et al. A systematic review of the effect of oral antioxidants on male infertility. *Reprod Biomed Online* 2010;20:711-723.
33. Tremellen K. Oxidative stress and male infertility –a clinical perspective. *Hum Reprod Update* 2008;14:243-258.
34. Safarinejad MR, Safarinejad S, Shafiei N, Safarinejad S.

Effects of the reduced form of coenzyme q(10) (ubiquinol) on semen parameters in men with idiopathic infertility: a double-blind, placebo controlled, randomized study. *J Urol* 2012;188:526-531.

35. Nadjarzadeh A, Shidfar F, Amirjannati N, et al. Effect of Coenzyme Q10 supplementation on antioxidant enzymes activity and oxidative stress of seminal plasma: a double-blind randomised clinical trial. *Andrologia* 2013;Epub ahead of print.

36. Mancini A, De Marinis L, Littarru G, et al. An update of Coenzyme Q10 implications in male infertility: biochemical and therapeutic aspects. *Biofactors* 2005;25:165-174.

Some content adapted from SpectraCell Laboratories, Inc.

Methylation

Methylation is the process during which a carbon and three hydrogen atoms are added to a molecule ($CH3^+$). This process participates in a variety of body functions, including detoxification of hormones, chemicals, and heavy metals; genetic expression and repair of DNA; energy production; and repair of cells damaged by free radicals.[1] Vitamins are essential for this process. Vitamin B2 (riboflavin), a precursor to FAD (Flavin adenine dinucleotide), helps to recycle folate (B9) into a usable methyl-donor form.[2-4] Folate is a methyl donor for many reactions in the body, including neurotransmitter synthesis and conversion of homocysteine to methionine. It is a precursor to SAMe (S-adenosylmethionine) and is also required for proper DNA synthesis.[5-7,15]

Vitamin B3 maintains proper methylation of genes that suppress tumor formation and growth.[8-10] Vitamin B6 is a cofactor for the enzyme—serine hydroxyl methyl transferase—that transfers methyl units[11,12] while Vitamin B12 is a vital enzyme needed in the synthesis of SAMe, the body's most important methyl donor. Methionine synthase, an enzyme that catalyzes the methylation cycle, is B12 dependent.[12-15] Choline is a major source of methyl groups (methyl donor), and a deficiency is linked to DNA damage.[16-18] Vitamin C deficiency alters methylation patterns in cancer cells and also is a cofactor for methylating enzymes.[19,20]

Several key enzymes needed for methylation reactions are copper dependent.[21-23] Interestingly, the role of magnesium in the methylation of genes that affect glucose metabolism may explain the co-occurrence between magnesium deficiency and diabetes.[24,25] Selenium inhibits a methylating enzyme (DNA methyltransferase) in cancer genes, effectively turning them off. Selenoproteins protect DNA and metabolize methionine.[26,27] A zinc deficiency can lower the ability to use methyl groups from methyl donors such as SAMe, thus causing global hypo-methylation of DNA.[28-30]

Two amino acids are significant for this process. Serine is an important methyl donor, especially in the case of a folate deficiency.[31-33] Glutathione deficiency impairs methylation reactions and impedes synthesis of the methyl donor SAMe.[34,36]

Reference List

1. Corey M. Methylation: *Why it matters for your immunity, inflammation and more.* http://www.mindbodygreen.com/0-18245/methylation-why-it-matters-for-your-immunity-inflammation-more.html. 9 Apr 2015. Accessed 16 Sep 2016.
2. Ames B, Elson-Schwab I, Silver E. High-dose vitamin therapy stimulates variant enzymes with decreased coenzyme binding affinity (increased K(m)): relevance to genetic disease and polymorphisms. *Am J Clin Nutr* 2002;75:616-658.
3. Dym I, Eisenberg D. Sequence-structure analysis of FAD-containing proteins. *Protein Sci* 2001;10:1712-1728.
4. Premkumar VG, Yuvaraj S, Shanthi P. Co-enzyme Q10, riboflavin and niacin supplementation on alteration of DNA repair enzyme and DNA methylation in breast cancer patients undergoing tamoxifen therapy. *Br J Nutr* 2008;100:1179-1182.
5. Miller A. The Methylation, Neurotransmitter, and Antioxidant Connections Between Folate and Depression. *Altern Med Rev* 2008;13:216-226.
6. Fenech M. Nutriomes and nutrient arrays - the key to personalised nutrition for DNA damage prevention and cancer growth control. *Genome Integr* 2010;1:11.
7. Moores CJ, Fenech M, O'Callaghan NJ. Telomere dynamics: the influence of folate and DNA methylation. *Ann NY Acad Sci* 2011;1229:76-88.
8. Hageman F, Stierum R. Niacin, poly(ADP-ribose) polymerase-1 and genomic stability. *Mutat Res* 2001;475:45-56.
9. Kang HT, Lee HI, Hwang ES. Nicotinamide extends replicative lifespan of human cells. *Aging Cell* 2006;5:423-436.
10. Kirkland JB. Niacin and carcinogenesis. *Nutr Cancer* 2003;46:110-118.
11. Davis C, Uthus E. DNA methylation, cancer susceptibility, and nutrient interactions. *Exp Biol Med* 2004;229:988-995.
12. Mashiyama S, Hansen C, Roitman E. An assay for uracil in human DNA at baseline: effect of marginal vitamin B6

deficiency. *Anal Biochem* 2008;372:21-31.

13. Ba Y, Yu H, Liu F, et al. Relationship of folate, vitamin B12 and methylation of insulin-like growth factor-II in maternal and cord blood. *Eur J Clin Nutr* 2011;65:480-485.

14. Das P, Singal R. DNA methylation and cancer. *J Clin Oncol* 2004;22:4632-4642.

15. Brunaud L, Alberto J, Ayav A, et al. Effects of vitamin B12 and folate deficiencies on DNA methylation and carcinogenesis in rat liver. *Clin Chem Lab Med* 2003;41:1012-1019.

16. da Costa, Niculescu M, Craciunescu C, et al. Choline deficiency increases lymphocyte apoptosis and DNA damage in humans. *Am J Clin Nutr* 2006;84:88-94.

17. Zeisel S. Nutritional genomics: defining the dietary requirement and effects of choline. *J Nutr* 2011;141:531-534.

18. Jiang X, Yan J, West A, et al. Maternal choline intake alters the epigenetic state of fetal cortisolregulating genes in humans. *FASEB J* 2012; Epub ahead of print.

19. Piyathilake C, Bell W, Johanning G, et al. The accumulation of ascorbic acid by squamous cell carcinomas of the lung and larynx is associated with global methylation of DNA. *Cancer* 2000;89:171-6

20. Chung T, Brena R, Kolle G, et al. Vitamin C promotes widespread yet specific DNA demethylation of the epigenome in human embryonic stem cells. *Stem Cells* 2010;28:1848-55.

21. Birkaya B, Aletta J. NGF promotes copper accumulation required for optimum neurite outgrowth and protein methylation. *J Neurobiol* 2005;63:49-61.

22. Winston G, Jaiser S. Copper deficiency myelopathy and subacute combined degeneration of the cord – why is the phenotype so similar? *Med Hypotheses* 2008;71:229-236.

23. Keen C, Hanna L, Lanoue L, et al. Developmental consequences of trace mineral deficiencies in rodents: acute and long-term effects. *J Nutr* 2003;133:1477S-1480S.

24. Takaya J, Iharada A, Okihana H, et al. Magnesium deficiency in pregnant rats atlers methylation of specific cytosines in the hepatic hydroxysteroid dehydrogenase-2 promoter of the offspring. *Epigenetics* 2011;6:573-578.

25. Huang y, Ji L, Huang Q, et al. Structural insights into

mechanisms of the small RNA methyltransfersase HEN1. *Nature* 2009;461:823-827.

26. Davis D, Uthus E, Finley J. Dietary selenium and arsenic affect DNA methylation in vitro in Caco-2 cells and in vivo in rat liver and colon. *J Nutr* 2000;130:2903-2909.

27. McCann J, Ames B. Adaptive dysfunction of selenoproteins from the perspective of the triage theory: why modest selenium deficiency may increase risk of diseases of aging. *FASEB J* 2011;25:1793-1814.

28. Sharif R, Thomas P, Zalewski P, Fenech M. The role of zinc in genomic stability. *Mutat Res* 2012;733:111-121.

29. Dresosti I. Zinc and the gene. *Mutat Res* 2001;475:161-167.

30. Wallwork J, Duerre J. Effect of zinc deficiency on methionine metabolism, methylation reactions and protein synthesis in isolated prefused rat liver. *J Nutr* 1985;115:252-262.

31. Kalhan S, Hanson R. Resurgence of serine: an often neglected but indispensable amino acid. *J Biol Chem* 2012;287:19786-91.

32. de Koning T, Snell K, et al. L-serine in disease and development. *Biochem J* 2003;371:653-661.

33. Townsend J, Davis S, Mackey A, et al. Folate deprivation reduces homocysteine remethylation in a human intestinal epithelial cell culture model: role of serine in one-carbon donation. *Am J Physiol Gastrointest Liver Physiol* 2004;286:G588-95.

34. Lertratanangkoon K, Wu CJ, Savaraj N, et al. Alterations of DNA methylation by glutathione depletion. *Cancer Lett* 1997;120:149-156.

35. Lee D, Jacobs D, Porta M. Hypothesis: a unifying mechanism for nutrition and chemicals as lifelong modulators of DNA hypomethylation. *Environ Health Perspect* 2009;117:1799-1802.

Some content adapted from SpectraCell Laboratories, Inc.

Neurology

Neurology is defined as that branch of medicine or biology that deals with the anatomy, functions, and organic disorders of nerves and the nervous system. While there are a variety of neurological disorders, only Alzheimer's, migraine headaches, multiple sclerosis, Parkinson's, and neuropathy are addressed in this section. In some studies, Vitamin B1 and Vitamin B12 have significantly reduced neuropathic pain.[1-3] Correcting deficiencies in B3, B6, B12 and folic acid (B9), may produce dramatic results for reducing the pain and frequency of migraine headaches.[4,5] Vitamin B2 also helps mitochondria (energy-producing centers in cells) to function properly.[6,7] Symptoms of multiple sclerosis (MS) are more severe when blood levels of Vitamin D are low, and research shows that over half of people with Parkinson's disease are deficient in Vitamin D.[8,9] Finally, a higher intake of Vitamin C and Vitamin E can slow the progression of dementia that is seen in Alzheimer's patients.[10]

Research shows that patients with MS have lowered calcium levels.[11] A copper deficiency can cause symptoms seen in MS patients as well.[12] Evidence confirms that a copper deficiency contributes to the progression of Alzheimer's disease.[13] A magnesium deficiency may be related to peripheral neuropathy: In one clinical study, oral doses of magnesium resulted in less pain for neuropathy.[14,15]

Much like the insulation that coats electronic wiring, nerves are covered with a protective coating called myelin. If the myelin sheath deteriorates, neurological problems arise, which is what happens to people with multiple sclerosis (MS). A vital enzyme needed to manufacture this protective coating contains serine, an important amino acid needed for neurological health. Consequently, a deficiency in this amino acid may be a contributing factor.[16] The pain reducing effects of carnitine, another amino acid,[17-18] and omega-3 fatty acids have been demonstrated in several studies.[19,20]

A high degree of oxidative stress at the cellular level could predispose a person to certain neurological complications. Antioxidant therapy has the potential to contribute to preventing or reduce many neurologic disorders. Supplementation with coenzyme Q10, a powerful antioxidant that aids energy metabolism, may lessen both the frequency and intensity of migraine headaches.[21,22] The role of oxidative stress in causing migraines is not totally understood, but studies do show that low levels of specific antioxidants, such as glutathione[23-25] and lipoic acid,[27] co-occur with migraine occurrence. High levels of oxidative stress increase neuropathic pain, which explains why the powerful antioxidants cysteine, Vitamin E, and lipoic acid may be successful in treating neuropathy.[26] Research also shows that the administration of coenzyme Q10 slows the neurological deterioration seen in Parkinson's disease.[28]

Reference List

1. Farvid MS, Homayouni F, Amiri Z, Adelmanesh F. Improving neuropathy scores in type 2 diabetic patients using micronutrients supplementation. *Diabetes Res Clin Pract.* 2011 Jul;93(1):86-94. doi: 10.1016/j.diabres.2011.03.016. Epub 2011 Apr 14. PMID: 21496936.
2. Rieder HP, Berger W, Fridrich R. Vitamin status in diabetic neuropathy (thiamine, riboflavin, pyridoxin, cobalamin and tocopherol. *Z Ernahrungswiss.* 1980 Mar;19(1):1-13. German. PMID: 7053098.
3. Talaei A, Siavash M, Majidi H, Chehrei A.Vitamin B12 may be more effective than nortriptyline in improving painful diabetic neuropathy. *Int J Food Sci Nutr.* 2009;60 Suppl 5:71-6. doi: 10.1080/09637480802406153. Epub 2009 Feb 11. PMID: 19212856.
4. Menon S, Lea RA, Ingle S, Sutherland M, Wee S, Haupt LM, Palmer M, Griffiths LR.Effects of dietary folate intake on migraine disability and frequency. *Headache.* 2015 Feb;55(2):301-9. doi: 10.1111/head.12490. Epub 2015 Jan 19. PMID: 25598270.
5. Shaik MM, Tan HL, Kamal MA, Gan SH. Do folate, vitamins B6 and B12 play a role in the pathogenesis of migraine? The role of pharmacoepigenomics. *CNS Neurol Disord Drug Targets.* 2014;13(5):828-35. Review. PMID: 24040787.
6. Henriques BJ, Lucas TG, Gomes CM. Therapeutic approaches using riboflavin in mitochondrial energy metabolism disorders. *Curr Drug Targets.* 2016 Aug 13. Epub ahead of print] PMID: 27527619.

7. Colombo B, Saraceno L, Comi G.Riboflavin and migraine: the bridge over troubled mitochondria. *Neurol Sci.* 2014 May;35 Suppl 1:141-4. doi: 10.1007/s10072-014-1755-z. PMID: 24867851.

8. Goodin DS. The epidemiology of multiple sclerosis: insights to a causal cascade. *Handb Clin Neurol.* 2016;138:173-206. doi: 10.1016/B978-0-12-802973-2.00011-2. PMID: 27637959.

9. Haas J, Schwarz A, Korporal-Kuhnke M, Faller S, Jarius S, Wildemann B.Hypovitaminosis D upscales B-cell immunoreactivity in multiple sclerosis. *J Neuroimmunol.* 2016 May 15;294:18-26. doi: 10.1016/j.jneuroim.2016.03.011. Epub 2016 Mar 23. PMID: 27138094.

10. Blaylock R. Excititoxins: The Taste That Kills. Santa Fe, NM: Health Press: 2011.

11. Schwarz A, Schumacher M, Pfaff D, et al.Fine-tuning of regulatory T cell function: the role of calcium signals and naive regulatory T cells for regulatory T cell deficiency in multiple sclerosis. *J Immunol.* 2013 May 15;190(10):4965-70. doi:10.4049/jimmunol.1203224. Epub 2013 Apr 10. PMID: 23576680.

12. Johnson S. The possible role of gradual accumulation of copper, cadmium, lead and iron and gradual depletion of zinc, magnesium, selenium, vitamins B2, B6, D, and E and essential fatty acids in multiple sclerosis. *Med Hypotheses.* 2000 Sep;55(3):239-41. PMID: 10985916.

13. Xu J, Begley P, Church SJ, Patassini S, et al. Elevation of brain glucose and polyol-pathway intermediates with accompanying brain-copper deficiency in patients with Alzheimer's disease: metabolic basis for dementia. *Sci Rep.* 2016 Jun 9;6:27524. doi: 10.1038/srep27524. PMID: 27276998.

14. Durlach J, Bac P, Durlach V, Bara M, Guiet-Bara A. Neurotic, neuromuscular and autonomic nervous form of magnesium imbalance. *Magnes Res.* 1997 Jun;10(2):169-95. Review. English, French. PMID: 9368238.

15. Yousef AA, Al-deeb AE. A double-blinded randomised controlled study of the value of sequential intravenous and oral magnesium therapy in patients with chronic low back

pain with a neuropathic component. *Anaesthesia.* 2013 Mar;68(3):260-6. doi: 10.1111/anae.12107. Epub 2012 Dec 17. PMID: 23384256.

16. Damseh N, Simonin A, Jalas C, et al. Mutations in SLC1A4, encoding the brain serine transporter, are associated with developmental delay, microcephaly and hypomyelination. *J Med Genet.* 2015 Aug;52(8):541-7. doi: 10.1136/jmedgenet-2015-103104. Epub 2015 Jun 3.PMID: 26041762.

17. Di Cesare Mannelli L, Ghelardini C, Calvani M, et al. Protective effect of acetyl-L-carnitine on the apoptotic pathway of peripheral neuropathy. *Eur J Neurosci.* 2007 Aug;26(4):820-7. PMID: 17714181.

18. Flatters SJ, Xiao WH, Bennett GJ. Acetyl-L-carnitine prevents and reduces paclitaxel-induced painful peripheral neuropathy. *Neurosci Lett.* 2006 Apr 24;397(3):219-23. Epub 2006 Jan 6. PMID: 16406309.

19. Yee P[1], Weymouth AE, Fletcher EL, Vingrys AJ. The role of omega-3 polyunsaturated fatty acid supplements in diabetic neuropathy. *Invest Ophthalmol Vis Sci.* 2010 Mar;51(3):1755-64. doi: 10.1167/iovs.09-3792. Epub 2009 Nov 11.

20. Dyuizen IV, Manzhulo IV, Ogurtsova OS, et al. Specific features of analgesic effect of docosahexaenoic acid in rats with neuropathic pain syndrome. *Bull Exp Biol Med.* 2014 Mar;156(5):699-701. doi: 10.1007/s10517-014-2428-x. Epub 2014 Mar 25. Erratum in: *Bull Exp Biol Med.* 2014 Apr;156(6):885. PMID: 24770761.

21. Gaul C, Diener HC, Danesch U; Migravent® Study Group. Improvement of migraine symptoms with a proprietary supplement containing riboflavin, magnesium and Q10: a randomized, placebo-controlled, double-blind, multicenter trial. *J Headache Pain.* 2015;16:516. doi: 10.1186/s10194-015-0516-6. Epub 2015 Apr 3. PMID: 25916335.

22. Slater SK, Nelson TD, Kabbouche MA, et al.A randomized, double-blinded, placebo-controlled, crossover, add-on study of CoEnzyme Q10 in the prevention of pediatric and adolescent migraine. *Cephalalgia.* 2011 Jun;31(8):897-905. doi: 10.1177/0333102411406755. Epub 2011 May 17. PMID: 21586650.

23. Kusumi M, Ishizaki K, Kowa H, et al. Glutathione S-transferase polymorphisms: susceptibility to migraine without aura. *Neurol.* 2003;49(4):218-22. PMID: 12736537.
24. Mattsson P, Bjelfman C, Lundberg PO, Rane A. Cytochrome P450 2D6 and glutathione S-transferase M1 genotypes and migraine. *Eur J Clin Invest.* 2000 Apr;30(4):367-71. PMID: 10759887.
25. Eren Y, Dirik E, Neşelioğlu S, Erel Ö. Oxidative stress and decreased thiol level in patients with migraine: cross-sectional study. *Acta Neurol Belg.* 2015 Dec;115(4):643-9. doi: 10.1007/s13760-015-0427-y. Epub 2015 Jan 17. PMID: 25595415.
26. Duggett NA, Griffiths LA, McKenna OE, et al. Oxidative stress in the development, maintenance and resolution of paclitaxel-induced painful neuropathy. *Neuroscience.* 2016 Oct 1;333:13-26. doi: 10.1016/j.neuroscience.2016.06.050. Epub 2016 Jul 5. PMID: 27393249.
27. Maglione E, Marrese C, Migliaro E, et al. Increasing bioavailability of (R)-alpha-lipoic acid to boost antioxidant activity in the treatment of neuropathic pain. *Acta Biomed.* 2015 Dec 14;86(3):226-33. PMID: 26694149.
28. Wu SS, Frucht SJ. Treatment of Parkinson's disease : what's on the horizon? *CNS Drugs.* 2005;19(9):723-43. Review. PMID: 16142989.

Some content adapted from SpectraCell Laboratories, Inc.

Obesity

Obesity is regarded as a chronic medical disease with serious health implications. The worldwide incidence of obesity more than doubled between 1980 and 2014. Obesity contributes to noncommunicable diseases, such as heart disease and stroke, diabetes, osteoarthritis, and some cancers.[1] Since adipose tissue (fat cells) has its own nutritional requirements, fat cells draw from nutritional reserves in much the same way other organs do in order to perform normal cellular functions. The combination of reduced bioavailability and increased demand for nutrients caused by excess adipose tissue ultimately causes multiple deficiencies that need to be addressed.

Blood vessels in overweight individuals are typically not as pliable and healthy as normal weight people due to various interrelated physiologic factors. Vitamin C supplementation has been demonstrated to improve vascular function in overweight people.[2] Obesity often reduces the bioavailability of certain nutrients, for example, D.[3] The effectiveness of Vitamin D supplementation is largely dependent on how overweight a person is.[4] Obese patients often need higher doses to attain Vitamin D repletion compared to individuals with normal body weight.[5] In a recent study, over 50% of obese patients were evaluated for Vitamin D status and found to be deficient.[6]

Studies with animals indicate that a form of Vitamin E (tocotrienol) inhibits pre-fat cells from changing into mature fat cells, resulting in a reduction in body fat.[7] Vitamin K supplementation can decrease the progression of insulin resistance since vitamin K dependent proteins are present in liver and pancreas, two organs essential for proper glucose (sugar) metabolism.[8,9]

Niacin (Vitamin B3) treatment has been shown to increase levels of adiponectin, a beneficial enzyme that regulates metabolism of glucose and fatty acids.[10,11] Reduced adiponectin levels co-occur with obesity and heart disease. In a similar study, Vitamin B5 raised the activity of lipoprotein lipase, an enzyme that helps breaks down fat cells so they can be processed by the body.[12] Other B Vitamins play an important role in the regulation of sugar and fat metabolism, which ultimately helps weakens insulin resistance. Riboflavin (Vitamin B2) helps metabolize food into energy.[13] A deficiency in Vitamin B6 can create glucose intolerance, and biotin is necessary for the proper metabolism of fats and carbohydrates.[14] In recent studies, the combination of chromium and biotin supplementation significantly enhanced glycemic control in overweight patients.[15-18]

The mineral chromium is a cofactor in the major hormone necessary for proper sugar metabolism. Recent studies have shown that chromium deficiency could negatively affect the ability to burn glucose effectively, thus contributing to a pre-diabetic or obese state. Epidemiological studies have reported that low zinc status is associated with a higher incidence of obesity. In fact, one animal study reported that zinc deficiency in mothers contributes to an expansion of body fat of their offspring.[19] This result may be due, in part, to the relationship between zinc and leptin, a beneficial hormone that regulates appetite. Zinc depletion diminishes leptin levels while restoring zinc reverses this effect.[20-22]

Calcium intake has also been associated with weight loss through its ability to inhibit the formation of fat cells. It also promotes the oxidation, or burning, of fat cells, therefore decreasing the risk of obesity.[23,24] Other minerals are necessary for proper insulin function as well, and deficiencies are common in overweight people. For example, a copper deficiency can impair glucose metabolism and strengthen insulin resistance.[25,26] The minerals magnesium, zinc, calcium and copper have all shown positive effects on blood pressure (see hypertension) and vascular health.

As with many other conditions, amino acids are a necessity for prevention and restoration of a healthy state. Carnitine is an important amino acid that helps muscle cells utilize energy and burn calories. Evidence shows that supplementation with carnitine when combined with an exercise program may create positive changes in body composition by decreasing visceral adiposity (belly fat) more efficiently than without supplementation.[27-28] Another amino acid, glutamine, has been shown to decrease fat mass and enhance glucose uptake in skeletal muscle. This consequently reduces insulin resistance, a major risk factor that contributes to obesity. Supplementation of the relatively unknown amino acid asparagine can improve insulin sensitivity by boosting the amount of sugar that muscle tissues consume to be burned for fuel. Asparagine also increases the capacity of muscles to utilize fatty acids for fuel, thus contributing to more efficient energy production and reduced obesity.[29,30]

Obesity severely damages the body's ability to efficiently

burn dietary carbohydrates. This is caused primarily by the body's inability to use insulin, the hormone that transports sugars into muscles where they can be used for fuel instead of being stored as fat. Lipoic acid has been shown to increase the rate of glucose consumption by muscle cells, which helps a person burn sugars more efficiently.[31,32] Numerous studies show a link between oxidative stress and inflammation with obesity. Visceral adiposity (fat around the belly) is particularly high in dangerous enzymes that cause oxidative stress.[33,34] Weight loss certainly thwarts this phenomenon, and studies show that the amount of weight loss directly correlates to decreases in oxidative stress. Since oxidative stress contributes to inflammation and inflammation causes oxidative stress, it is vitally important that antioxidant status be optimized, especially in the obese patient.[35,36]

Visceral adiposity also causes inflammation of the liver (known as fatty liver), which is particularly common in obese people One recent study demonstrated that coenzyme Q10 reduced obesity-induced inflammation of the liver.[37] Similarly, inflammation in blood vessels of obese patients contributes to heart disease and stroke, which can be alleviated in part through proper antioxidant supplementation.

Overweight people tend to have high blood pressure (see hypertension), worsened by vitamin deficiencies. Since so many nutrients (folate, biotin, carnitine, Vitamins A, C, E and several minerals) are involved in the maintenance of healthy blood vessels of both normal weight and overweight people, a comprehensive evaluation of how they are performing in the cells of obese patients is invaluable.

Reference List

1. World Health Organization. *Obesity and overweight.* http://www.who.int/mediacentre/factsheets/fs311/en/. June 2016. Accessed 16 Sep 2016.
2. de Sousa MG, Yugar-Toledo JC, Rubira M, Ferreira-Melo SE, et al. Ascorbic acid improves impaired venous and arterial endothelium-dependent dilation in smokers. *Acta Pharmacol Sin.* 2005 Apr;26(4):447-52. PMID:15780194.
3. Karonova T, Belyaeva O, Jude EB, et al. Serum 25(OH)D and adipokines levels in people with abdominal obesity. *J*

Steroid Biochem Mol Biol. 2016 Sep 11. pii: S0960-0760(16)30241-2. doi: 10.1016/j.jsbmb.2016.09.005. [Epub ahead of print] Review. PMID: 27629594.

4. Abbas MA. Physiological functions of Vitamin D in adipose tissue. *J Steroid Biochem Mol Biol.* 2016 Aug 9. pii: S0960-0760(16)30219-9. doi: 10.1016/j.jsbmb.2016.08.004. Epub ahead of print. Review. PMID: 27520301.

5. De Souza Silva J, Pereira SE, Saboya Sobrinho CJ, Ramalho A. Obesity, related diseases and their relationship with vitamin D deficiency in adolescents. *Nutr Hosp.* 2016 Jul 19;33(4):381. doi: 10.20960/nh.381. PMID: 27571659.

6. Vogt S, Baumert J, Peters A, Thorand B, Scragg R. Effect of waist circumference on the association between serum 25-hydroxyvitamin D and serum lipids: results from the National Health and Nutrition Examination Survey 2001-2006. *Public Health Nutr.* 2016 Jul 29:1-10. [Epub ahead of print] PMID: 27469173.

7. Zhao L, Fang X, Marshall MR, Chung S. Regulation of Obesity and Metabolic Complications by Gamma and Delta Tocotrienols. *Molecules.* 2016 Mar 11;21(3):344. doi: 10.3390/molecules21030344. Review. PMID: 26978344.

8. Manna P, Kalita J. Beneficial role of vitamin K supplementation on insulin sensitivity, glucose metabolism, and the reduced risk of type 2 diabetes: A review. *Nutrition.* 2016 Jul-Aug;32(7-8):732-9. doi: 10.1016/j.nut.2016.01.011. Epub 2016 Jan 25. Review. PMID: 27133809.

9. Choi HJ, Yu J, Choi H, et al. Vitamin K2 supplementation improves insulin sensitivity via osteocalcin metabolism: a placebo-controlled trial. *Diabetes Care.* 2011 Sep;34(9):e147. doi: 10.2337/dc11-0551. No abstract available. PMID: 21868771.

10. Hu M, Yang YL, Masuda D, Yamashita S, Tomlinson B. Effect of Extended-Release Niacin/Laropiprant Combination on Plasma Adiponectin and Insulin Resistance in Chinese Patients with Dyslipidaemia. *Dis Markers.* 2015;2015:154014. doi: 10.1155/2015/154014. Epub 2015 Apr 29. PMID: 26063948.

11. Wanders D, Graff EC, White BD, Judd RL. Niacin increases adiponectin and decreases adipose tissue

inflammation in high fat diet-fed mice. *PLoS One.* 2013 Aug 13;8(8):e71285. doi: 10.1371/journal.pone.0071285. eCollection 2013. PMID: 23967184.

12. Naruta E, Buko V. Hypolipidemic effect of pantothenic acid derivatives in mice with hypothalamic obesity induced by aurothioglucose. *Exp Toxicol Pathol.* 2001 Oct;53(5):393-8.

13. Henriques BJ, Lucas TG, Gomes CM. Therapeutic approaches using riboflavin in mitochondrial energy metabolism disorders. *Curr Drug Targets.* 2016 Aug 13. [Epub ahead of print] PMID: 27527619.

14. Adams PW, Wynn V, Folkard J, Seed M. Influence of oral contraceptives, pyridoxine (vitamin B6), and tryptophan on carbohydrate metabolism. *Lancet.* 1976 Apr 10;1(7963):759-64. PMID: 56585.

15. Albarracin C, Fuqua B, Geohas J, et al. Combination of chromium and biotin improves coronary risk factors in hypercholesterolemic type 2 diabetes mellitus: a placebo-controlled, double-blind randomized clinical trial. *J Cardiometab Syndr.* 2007 Spring;2(2):91-7.PMID:17684468.

16. Geohas J, Daly A, Juturu V, Finch M, Komorowski JR. Chromium picolinate and biotin combination reduces atherogenic index of plasma in patients with type 2 diabetes mellitus: a placebo-controlled, double-blinded, randomized clinical trial. *Am J Med Sci.* 2007 Mar;333(3):145-53. PMID: 17496732.

17. Singer GM, Geohas J. The effect of chromium picolinate and biotin supplementation on glycemic control in poorly controlled patients with type 2 diabetes mellitus: a placebo-controlled, double-blinded, randomized trial. *Diabetes Technol Ther.* 2006 Dec;8(6):636-43. PMID: 17109595

18. Fuhr JP Jr, He H, Goldfarb N, Nash DB. Use of chromium picolinate and biotin in the management of type 2 diabetes: an economic analysis. *Dis Manag.* 2005 Aug;8(4):265-75. PMID: 16117721.

19. Padmavathi IJ, Kishore YD, Venu L, Ganeshan M, Harishankar N, Giridharan NV, Raghunath M. Prenatal and perinatal zinc restriction: effects on body composition, glucose tolerance and insulin response in rat offspring. *Exp*

Physiol. 2009 Jun;94(6):761-9. doi: 10.1113/expphysiol.2008.045856. Epub 2009 Feb 27.

20. García OP, Long KZ, Rosado JL. Impact of micronutrient deficiencies on obesity. *Nutr Rev.* 2009 Oct;67(10):559-72. doi: 10.1111/j.1753-4887.2009.00228.x. Review. PMID: 19785688.

21. Chen MD. Hyper- or hypoleptinemia in subjects with zinc deficiency? *J Med Food.* 2005 Spring;8(1):117-8; author reply 118-9. No abstract available. PMID:15857222.

22. Mantzoros CS, Prasad AS, Beck FW, et al. Zinc may regulate serum leptin concentrations in humans. *J Am Coll Nutr.* 1998 Jun;17(3):270-5. PMID: 9627914.

23. Booth AO, Huggins CE, Wattanapenpaiboon N, Nowson CA. Effect of increasing dietary calcium through supplements and dairy food on body weight and body composition: a meta-analysis of randomised controlled trials. *Br J Nutr.* 2015 Oct 14;114(7):1013-25. doi: 10.1017/S0007114515001518. Epub 2015 Aug 3. Review. PMID: 26234296.

24. Zhu W, Cai D, Wang Y, et al. Calcium plus vitamin D3 supplementation facilitated fat loss in overweight and obese college students with very-low calcium consumption: a randomized controlled trial. *Nutr J.* 2013 Jan 8;12:8. doi: 10.1186/1475-2891-12-8. Erratum in: *Nutr J.* 2013;12:43. PMID: 23297844.

25. Rosario JF, Gomez MP, Anbu P. Does the maternal micronutrient deficiency (copper or zinc or vitamin E) modulate the expression of placental 11 beta hydroxysteroid dehydrogenase-2 per se predispose offspring to insulin resistance and hypertension in later life? *Indian J Physiol Pharmacol.* 2008 Oct-Dec;52(4):355-65. PMID: 19585752.

26. Obeid O, Elfakhani M, Hlais S, et al. Plasma copper, zinc, and selenium levels and correlates with metabolic syndrome components of lebanese adults. *Biol Trace Elem Res.* 2008 Summer;123(1-3):58-65. doi: 10.1007/s12011-008-8112-0. Epub 2008 Feb 21. PMID: 18288450.

27. Hongu N, Sachan DS. Caffeine, carnitine and choline supplementation of rats decreases body fat and serum leptin concentration as does exercise. *J Nutr.* 2000 Feb;130(2):152-7. PMID: 10720162.

---

28. Stephens FB, Wall BT, Marimuthu K, et al. Skeletal muscle carnitine loading increases energy expenditure, modulates fuel metabolism gene networks and prevents body fat accumulation in humans. *J Physiol.* 2013 Sep 15;591(18):4655-66. doi: 10.1113/jphysiol.2013.255364. Epub 2013 Jul 1. PMID: 23818692.

29. Prada PO, Hirabara SM, de Souza CT, et al. L-glutamine supplementation induces insulin resistance in adipose tissue and improves insulin signalling in liver and muscle of rats with diet-induced obesity. *Diabetologia.* 2007 Sep;50(9):1949-59. Epub 2007 Jun 29.

30. Bierczyńska-Krzysik A, Łopaciuk M, Pawlak-Morka R, Stadnik D. Investigation of asparagine deamidation in a SOD1-based biosynthetic human insulin precursor by MALDI-TOF mass spectrometry. *Acta Biochim Pol.* 2014;61(2):349-57. Epub 2014 Jun 16. PMID: 24936522.

31. Lancha AH Jr, Poortmans JR, Pereira LO. The effect of 5 days of aspartate and asparagine supplementation on glucose transport activity in rat muscle. *Cell Biochem Funct.* 2009 Dec;27(8):552-7. doi: 10.1002/cbf.1606. PMID:19821260.

32. Estrada DE, Ewart HS, Tsakiridis T, et al. Stimulation of glucose uptake by the natural coenzyme alpha-lipoic acid/thioctic acid: participation of elements of the insulin signaling pathway. *Diabetes.* 1996 Dec;45(12):1798-804. PMID: 8922368.

33. Wang Y, Li X, Guo Y, Chan L, Guan X. Alpha-Lipoic acid increases energy expenditure by enhancing adenosine monophosphate-activated protein kinase-peroxisome proliferator-activated receptor-gamma coactivator-1alpha signaling in the skeletal muscle of aged mice. *Metabolism.* 2010 Jul;59(7):967-76. doi: 10.1016/j.metabol.2009.10.018. Epub 2009 Dec 16.PMID: 20015518.

34. Kuzmenko DI, Udintsev SN, Klimentyeva TK, Serebrov VY. Oxidative stress in adipose tissue as a primary link in pathogenesis of insulin resistance. *Biomed Khim.* 2016 Jan-Feb;62(1):14-21. doi: 10.18097/PBMC20166201014. Review. Russian. PMID: 26973182.

35. Liu R, Pulliam DA, Liu Y, Salmon AB. Dynamic differences in oxidative stress and the regulation of metabolism with age in visceral versus subcutaneous adipose. *Redox Biol.* 2015

Dec;6:401-8. doi: 10.1016/j.redox.2015.07.014. Epub 2015 Sep 3. PMID: 26355396.

36. Farsi F, Mohammadshahi M, Alavinejad P,et al.Functions of Coenzyme Q10 Supplementation on Liver Enzymes, Markers of Systemic Inflammation, and Adipokines in Patients Affected by Nonalcoholic Fatty Liver Disease: A Double-Blind, Placebo-Controlled, Randomized Clinical Trial. *J Am Coll Nutr.* 2016 May-Jun;35(4):346-53. doi: 10.1080/07315724.2015.1021057. Epub 2015 Jul 9. PMID: 26156412.

Some content adapted from SpectraCell Laboratories, Inc.

Pain

As of 2015, fifty million people reported significant or chronic pain. Ethnicity and gender played a role in reporting of pain with women, older people, and non-Hispanics more likely to report pain and Asian Americans less likely to report pain.[1] Nearly four times as many people suffer from chronic pain than diabetes.[2] The importance of micronutrient deficiencies cannot be underestimated in incidences of chronic pain.

As with many conditions, deficiencies in B Vitamins are a contributing factor. In animal studies, treatment with inositol induces antinociception (pain reduction).[3,4] Choline activates specific receptors in brain and spine that lower acute pain.[5,6] Vitamins B1, B2, B6, and B12 produce a dose dependent decrease in various kinds of pain (heat, pressure, chemical). In other words, how much pain reduction is achieved is related to the amount of the dosage of B Vitamins. These vitamins increase the sensitivity to pain meds, and their effect is likely mediated through serotonergic neurotransmitters.[7-10] A Vitamin D deficiency often presents clinically as muscle or bone pain.[11-13] Vitamin E reduces neuropathic pain,[14] and Vitamin C can lower morphine consumption after surgery.[15]

The presence of sufficient quantities of minerals can reduce pain. Magnesium lowers pain by blocking NMDA (N-methyl-D-aspartate) receptors in spinal cord, and it is effective in reducing post-operative pain.[16-18] Minerals are a cofactor for the powerful antioxidant super oxide dismutase that fights free radicals, a known source of pain. Copper supplementation can relieve arthritic pain. Treatment with selenium improves muscle pain in deficient patients. Research suggests both zinc and calcium play a role in the transmission of pain signals through nerves.[19-22]

Certain amino acids can help with pain. Cysteine reduces pain caused by systemic inflammation due to its potent antioxidant properties.[23,24] A deficiency of carnitine may exhibit itself as muscle weakness, pain (myalgia), or neuropathy. Supplementation reduces several types of chronic pain.[25-27] Lipoic acid is a very effective treatment for neuropathic pain.[28,29] Clinical trials show antioxidant therapy is an effective treatment for chronic pain. Coenzyme Q10 relieves statin-induced myopathy and neuropathy.[13,14,30-32] Oleic acid, a fatty acid found in olive oil and nuts, is a precursor of oleamide, an analgesic that affects neurotransmitters such as dopamine, serotonin, acetylcholine and GABA (gamma amino butyric acid). All of these play a role in pain signaling.[33,34]

Reference List

1. Weber C. *NIH study shows prevalence of chronic or severe pain in U.S. adults.* http://americanpainsociety.org/about-us/press-room/nih-study-shows-prevalence-of-chronic-or-severe-pain-in-u-s-adults. 18 Aug 2015. Accessed 16 Sep 2016.
2. American Academcy of Pain Medicine. *AAPM facts and figures on pain.* ww.painmed.org/patientcenter/facts_on_pain.aspx. Accessed 16 Sep 2016.
3. Shaldubina A, Buccafusca R, Johanson R, et al. Behavioural phenotyping of sodium-myo-inositol cotransporter heterozygous knockout mice with reduced brain inositol. *Genes Brain Behav* 2007;6:253-259.
4. Hamurtekin E, Gurun M. The antinociceptive effects of centrally administered CDP-choline on acute pain models in rats: the involvement of cholinergic system. *Brain Res* 2006;1117:92-100.
5. Wang Y, Su D, Wang R, et al. Antinociceptive effects of choline against acute and inflammatory pain. *Neuroscience* 2005;132:49-56.
6. Bertollo C, Oliveira A, Rocha L, et al. Characterization of the antinociceptive and anti-inflammatory activities of riboflavin in different experimental models. *Eur J Pharmacol* 2006;547:184-191.
7. Caram-Salas N, Reyes-Garcia G, Medina-Santillan R, et al. Thiamine and cyanocobalamin relieve neuropathic pain in rats: synergy with dexamethasone. *Pharmacology* 2006;77:53-62.
8. Wang Z, Gan Q, Rupert R, et al. Thiamine, pyridoxine, cyanocobalamin and their combination inhibit thermal, but not mechanical hyperalgesia in rats with primary sensory neuron injury. *Pain* 2005;114:266-277.
9. Bartoszyk G, Wild A. Antinociceptive effects of pyridoxine, thiamine, and cyanocobalamin in rats. *Ann NY Acad Sci*

1990;585:473-476.

10. Turner M, Hooten W, Schmidt J, et al. Prevalence and Clinical Correlates of Vitamin D Inadequacy among Patients with Chronic Pain. *Pain Med* 2008;9:979-984.

11. Mascarenhas R, Mobarhan S. Hypovitaminosis D-induced pain. *Nutr Rev* 2004;62:354-359.

12. Plotnikoff G, Quigley J. Prevalence of severe hypovitaminosis D in patients with persistent, nonspecific musculoskeletal pain. *Mayo Clin Proc* 2003;78:1463-1470.

13. Kim H, Kim J, Gao X, et al. Analgesic effect of vitamin E is mediated by reducing central sensitization in neuropathic pain. *Pain* 2006;122:53-62.

14. Kanazi G, El-Khatib M, Yazbeck-Karam V, et al. Effect of vitamin C on morphine use after laparoscopic cholecystectomy: a randomized controlled trial. *Can J Anaesth* 2012;59:538-543.

15. Arcioni R, Palmisani S, Tigano S, et al. Combined intrathecal and epidural magnesium sulfate supplementation of spinal anesthesia to reduce post-operative analgesic requirements: a prospective, randomized, double-blind, controlled trial in patients undergoing major orthopedic surgery. *Acta Anaesthesiol Scand* 2007;51:482-489.

16. Lysakowski C, Dumont L, Czarnetzki C, et al. Magnesium as an adjuvant to postoperative analgesia: a systematic review of randomized trials. *Anesth Analg* 2007;104:1532-1539.

17. Alloui A, Begon S, Chassaing C, et al. Does Mg2+ deficiency induce a long-term sensitization of the central nociceptive pathways? *Eur J Pharmacol* 2003;469:65-69.

18. Arisan E, Arisan S, Kiremit M, et al. Manganese superoxide dismutase polymorphism in chronic pelvic pain syndrome patients. *Prostate Cancer Prostatic Dis* 2006;9:426-431.

19. DiSilvestro R, Marten J, Skehan M. Effects of copper supplementation on ceruloplasmin and copeer-zinc superoxide dismutase in free-living rheumatoid arthritis patients. *J Am Coll Nutr* 1992;11:177-180.

20. Chariot P, Bignani O. Skeletal muscle disorders associated with selenium deficiency in humans. *Muscle Nerve* 2003;27:662-668.

21. Jo S, Danscher G, Schroder H, et al. Depletion of vesicular zinc in dorsal horn of spinal cord causes increased

---

neuropathic pain in mice. *Biometals* 2008;21:151-158.
22. Galeotti N, Bartolini A, Ghelardini C. Role of intracellular calcium in acute thermal pain perception. *Neuropharmacology* 2004;47:935-944.
23. Schmidtko A, Gao W, Sausbier M, et al. Cysteine-rich protein 2, a novel downstream effector ofcGMP/cGMP-dependent protein kinase I-mediated persistent inflammatory pain. *J Neurosci* 2008;28:1320-1330.
24. Pathirathna S, Covey D, Todorovic S, et al. Differential effects of endogenous cysteine analogs on peripheral thermal nociception in intact rats. *Pain* 2006;125:53-64.
25. Sima A, Calvani M, Mehra M, et al. Acetyl-L-carnitine improves pain, nerve regeneration, and vibratory perception in patients with chronic diabetic neuropathy: an analysis of two randomized placebo-controlled trials. *Diabetes Care* 2005;28:89-94.
26. Rossini M, Di Munno O, Valentini G, et al. Double-blind, multicenter trial comparing acetyl l-carnitine with placebo in the treatment of fibromyalgia patients. *Clin Exp Rheumatol* 2007;25:182-188.
27. Sima A. Acetyl-L-carnitine in diabetic polyneuropathy: experimental and clinical data. *CNS Drugs* 2007;21 Suppl 1:13-23:discussion 45-46.
28. Kirk G, White J, McKie L, et al. Combined antioxidant therapy reduces pain and improves quality of life in chronic pancreatitis. *J Gastrointest Surg* 2006;10:499-503.
29. Viggiano A, Monda M, Viggiano D, et al. Trigeminal pain transmission requires reactive oxygen species production. *Brain Res* 2005;1050:72-78.
30. Kim H, Kim J, Gao X, et al. Analgesic effect of vitamin E is mediated by reducing central sensitization in neuropathic pain. *Pain* 2006;122:53-62.
31. Kanazi G, El-Khatib M, Yazbeck-Karam V, et al. Effect of vitamin C on morphine use after laparoscopic cholecystectomy: a randomized controlled trial. *Can J Anaesth* 2012;59:538-543.
32. Marcoff L, Thompson P. The role of coenzyme Q10 in statin-associated myopathy: a systematic review. *J Am Coll Cardiol* 2007;49:2231-2237.
33. Mueller G, Driscoll W. Biosynthesis of oleamide. *Vitam*

Horm 2009;81:55-78.

34. Akanmu M, Adeosun S, Ilesanmi O. Neuropharmalogical effects of oleamide in male and female mice. *Behav Brain Res* 2007;182:88-94.

Some content adapted from SpectraCell Laboratories, Inc.

Sleep Apnea

Sleep apnea affects an estimated twenty-five million people in the U.S. It is associated with increased risk for high blood pressure, heart disease, Type 2 diabetes, stroke, and depression.[1] Vitamin C improves endothelial function (blood vessel health) in sleep apnea patients to levels seen in people without sleep apnea.[2-4] Vitamin E mitigates the oxidative stress seen in sleep apnea patients and works synergistically with Vitamin C.[5-7] Sleep apnea patients have low retinol (Vitamin A). Retinol suppresses the growth of vascular smooth muscle, an activity that causes blood vessels to clog, consequently linking low Vitamin A levels to the cardiovascular complications seen in sleep apnea patients.[8,9] People with sleep apnea have a high prevalence of Vitamin D deficiency. The worse the apnea the more severe is the nutritional deficiency. The evidence suggests low Vitamin D worsens the risk of heart disease created by sleep apnea.[10-12]

The importance of mineral supplementation cannot be underestimated. In one report, selenium supplementation completely stopped snoring caused by non-obesity sleep apnea. The role of selenium as a powerful antioxidant may decrease the oxidative stress seen in sleep apnea patients.[13-15] Copper is considered a strong predictor of oxidative stress in sleep apnea patients. The role of copper as a vital cofactor in the potent antioxidant superoxide dismutase (SOD) explains this. SOD is very low in apnea patients.[16,17] The trace minerals zinc, copper, magnesium, manganese and selenium are critical cofactors for the major antioxidant enzymes that are important in repairing cellular damage caused by hypoxia (lack of oxygen) in sleep apnea.[18,19]

Supplementation of certain amino acids and antioxidants is necessary. Oral supplementation with cysteine, the precursor to glutathione, has therapeutic potential for sleep apnea. Snore time and duration were significantly reduced for patients treated with N-acetyl cysteine compared to untreated sleep apnea patients.[20-21] Sleep apnea patients have both decreased anti-oxidant capacity and higher levels of oxidative stress than those in control groups.[7,23-25] Low levels of glutathione co-occur with sleep apnea. This powerful antioxidant also helps repair liver damage caused by sleep apnea.[26-28]

Reference List

1. National Healthy Sleep Awareness Project. *Rising prevalence of sleep apnea in U.S. threatens public health.* http://www.aasmnet.org/articles.aspx?id=5043. 29 Sep 2014. Accessed 16 Sep 2016.

2. Grebe M, Eisele HJ, Weissmann N, et al. Antioxidant vitamin C improves endothelial function in obstructive sleep apnea. *Am J Respir Crit Care Med.* 2006;173:897-901.

3. Büchner NJ, Quack I, Woznowski M et al. Microvascular endothelial dysfunction in obstructive sleep apnea is caused by oxidative stress and improved by continuous positive airway pressure therapy. *Respiration* 2011;82:409-417.

4. Celec P, Jurkovicová I, Buchta R, et al. Antioxidant vitamins prevent oxidative and carbonyl stress in an animal model of obstructive sleep apnea. *Sleep Breath* 2012 June 7 [Epub ahead of print].

5. Singh T, Patial K, Vijayan K, et al. Oxidative stress and obstructive sleep apnoea syndrome. *Indian J Chest Dis Allied Sci* 2009;51:217-224.

6. Lee D, Badr M, Mateika J, et al. Progressive augmentation and ventilatory long-term facilitation are enhanced in sleep apnoea patients and are mitigated by antioxidant administration. *J Phsyiol* 2009;587:5451-5467.

7. Day R, Matus I, Suzuki Y, et al. Plasma levels of retinoids, carotenoids and tocopherols in patients with mild obstructive sleep apnea. *Respirology* 2009;14:1134-1142.

8. Barcelo A, Barbe F, de la Pena M, et al. Antioxidant status in patients with sleep apnoea and impact of continuous positive airway pressure treatment. *Eur Respir J* 2006;27:756-760.

9. Mete T, Yalcin Y, Berker D, et al. Obstructive sleep apnea syndrome and its association with Vitamin D deficiency. *J Endocrinol Invest* 2013 April [Epub ahead of print]

10. Bozkurt NC, Cakal E, Sahin M, et al. The relation of serum 25-hydroxyvitamin –D levels with severity of obstructive sleep apnea and glucose metabolism abnormalities. *Endocrine* 2012;41:518-525.

11. Barceló A, Esquinas C, Piérola J, et al. Vitamin D Status and Parathyroid Hormone Levels in Patients with Obstructive

Sleep Apnea. *Respiration* 2012 Nov 15. [Epub ahead of print]

12. Dekok H. Case report: the medical treatment of obstructive sleep apnoea syndrome (OSAS) with Selenium. *Med Hypotheses*. 2005;65:817-818.

13. Kato M, Roberts-Thompson P, Philips B, et al. Impairment of endothelial-dependent vasodilation of resistance vessels in patients with obstructive sleep apnea. *Circulation* 2000;102:2607-2610.

14. Schnabel R, Lubos E, Messow C, et al. Selenium supplementation improves antioxidant capacity in vitro and in vivo in patients with coronary artery disease. The Selenium Therapy in Coronary Artery Disease Patients (SETCAP) Study. *Am J Heart* 2008;156:1201e1-11.

15. Volná J, Kemlink D, Kalousová M, et al. Biochemical oxidative stress-related markers in patients with obstructive sleep apnea. *Med Sci Monit* 2011;17:CR491-7.

16. Wysocka E, Cofta S, Piorunek T, et al. Blood antoxidant status, dysglycemia and obstructive sleep apnea. *Adv Exp Med Biol* 2013;756:121-129.

17. Wysocka E, Cofta S, Cymerys M, et al. The ipact of the sleep apnea syndrome on oxidant-antioxidant balance in the blood of overweight and obese patients. *J Physiol Pharmaco*. 2008;59 Suppl 6:761-769.

18. Shan X, Chi L, Ke Y, et al. Manganese superoxide dismutase protects mouse cortical neurons from chronic intermittent hypoxia-mediated oxidative damage. *Neurobiol Dis* 2007;28:206-215.

19. Sadasivam K, Patial K, Vijayan V, et al. Anti-oxidant treatment in obstructive sleep apnoea syndrome. *Indian J Chest Dis Allied Sci* 2011;53:153-162.

20. Liu J, Zhang J, Lu G, et al. The effect of oxidative stress in myocardial cell injury in mice exposed to chronic intermttant hypoxia. *Chin Med J* 2010;123:74-78.

21. Sekhar R, Patel S, Guthikonia A, et al. Deficient synthesis of glutathione underles oxidative stress in aging and can be corrected by dietary cysteine and glycine supplementation. *Am J Clin Nutr* 2011;94:847-853.

22. Dunleavy M, Bradford A, O'Halloran K. Oxidative stress impairs upper airway muscle endurance in an animal model

---

of sleep-disordered breathing. *Adv Exp Med Biol* 2008;605:458-462.

23. Murri M, Garcia-Delgado R, Alcázar-Ramirez J, et al. Assessment of cellular and plasma oxidative 2010;56:397-406.

24. Baldwin C, Bootzin R, Schwenke D, et al. Antioxidant nutrient intake and supplements as potential moderators of cognitive decline and cardiovascular disease in obstructive sleep apnea. *Sleep Med Rev* 2005;9:459-476.

25. Katsoulis K, Kontakiotis T, Spanogiannis D, et al. Total antioxidant status in patients with obstructive sleep apnea without comorbidities: the role of the severity of the disease. *Sleep Breath.* 2011 Dec;15:861-866.

26. Rosa DP, Martinez D, Picada J, et al. Hepatic oxidative stress in an animal model of sleep apnoea: effects of different duration of exposure. *Comp Hepatol* 2011 Jul 5; 10 (1):1. doi: 10.1186/1476-5926-10-1.

27. Ntalapascha M, Makris D, Kyparos A, et al. Oxidative stress in patients with obstructive sleep apnea syndrome. *Sleep Breath* 2012 [Epub ahead of print]

28. Mancuso M, Bonanni E, LoGerfo A, et al. Oxidative stress biomarkers in patients with untreated obstructive sleep apnea syndrome. *Sleep Med* 2012;13:632-636.

Some content adapted from SpectraCell Laboratories, Inc.

Sports Nutrition

Growing numbers of people are involved in exercise. The athlete's nutritional focus should include protein for muscle rebuilding, carbohydrates for energy renewal, fats for nerve function as well as the critically important vitamins, minerals, antioxidants and amino acids.

Among the nutrients needed are vitamins. Vitamin C, required for collagen synthesis, decreases post-workout soreness and protects muscles from injury due to trauma or training. It decreases cortisol created muscle catabolism.[1-3] Intense training causes cellular stress, and Vitamin E protects the enzymes responsible for repairing this cellular damage.[4,5] Vitamin D enhances bone strength, which reduces potential for sports-related injuries and stress fractures.[6,7] B Vitamins are cofactors for efficient energy metabolism from food. Synthesizing red blood cells requires folate (B9) and B12. Deficiencies in various B Vitamins may slow healing in sports injuries.[8,9]

Minerals are also required. For example, zinc interacts with hormones to enhance body composition and strength. A zinc deficiency impairs peak oxygen uptake during exercise. Often low zinc is common in distance runners and gymnasts, so copper must accompany supplementation with zinc to maintain balance.[10-12] Magnesium is the key to the production of ATP (adenosine triphosphate), the body's main storage form of energy. Magnesium supplementation may increase aerobic performance and enhance muscle strength and repair.[13,14]

Cysteine, an amino acid, decreases time to fatigue in endurance sports such as cycling. Because it is a precursor to glutathione, its supplementation raises glutathione levels.[15-17] Serine, another amino acid, keeps an athlete's hormone profile healthy by buffering post-workout cortisol levels that can cause excess muscle breakdown. It may also increase aerobic capacity.[18-20] The amino acid asparagine increases the capacity of muscle to use fatty acids and spare glycogen, increasing time to physical exhaustion. Intensive training lowers asparagine levels.[21-23] Glutamine depletion compromises immunity in many athletes after intense physical training. Marathoners who had glutamine supplementation reduced post-race infections.[24-27]

The antioxidant coenzyme Q10 diminishes muscle damage

after high intensity training. Studies indicate CoQ10 benefits strength and endurance. Olympic athletes who took 300 mg of CoQ10 had increased power.[28-30] Lipoic acid decreases cellular damage due to intense physical exercise while it also recycles other antioxidants, such as glutathione[31,32] that is a powerful antioxidant that detoxifies cellular by-products after workouts. As a result, reduced blood levels of glutathione are counterproductive to an athlete in training.[33,34] Carnitine allows cells to use fatty acids as an efficient non-glycogen source of fuel and improves muscle recovery while offsetting the rise in creatinine kinase, an indicator of muscle damage.[35,36]

Reference List

1. Bryer S, Goldfarb A. Effect of high dose vitamin C supplementation on muscle soreness, damage, function, and oxidative stress to eccentric exercise. *Int J Sport Nutr Exerc Metab* 2006;16:270-280.
2. Thompson D, Williams C, McGregor S, et al. Prolonged vitamin C supplementation and recovery from demanding exercise. *Int J Sport Nutr Exerc Metab* 2001;11:466-481.
3. Nakhostin-Roohi B, Babaei P, Rahmani F, et al. Effect of vitamin C supplementation on lipid peroxidation, muscle damage and inflammation after 30-min exercise at 75% VO2 max. *J Sports Med Phys Fitness* 2008;48:217-224.
4. Tsakiris S, Karikas G, Parthimos T, et al. Alpha-tocopherol supplementation prevents the exercise-induced reduction of serum paraoxonase 1/arylesterase activities in healthy individuals. *Eur J Clin Nutr* 2009;63:215-221.
5. Naziroglu M, Kilinc F, Uguz A, et al. Oral vitamin C and E combination modulates blood lipid peroxidation and antioxidant vitamin levels in maximal exercising basketball players. *Cell Biochem Funct* 2010;28:300-305.
6. Ogan D, Pritchett K. Vitamin D and the athlete: risks, recommendations, and benefits. *Nutrient* 2013;5:1856-1868.
7. Lewis R, Redzic M, Thomas D. The effects of seaon-long vitamin D supplementation on collegiate swimmers and divers. *Int J Sport Nutr Exerc Metab* 2013 Epub ahead of print.
8. Woolf K, Manore M. B-vitamins and exercise: does exercise

alter requirements? *Int J Sport Nutr Exerc Metab* 2006;16:453-484.

9. Manore M. Effect of physical activity on thiamine, riboflavin and vitamin B6 requirements. *Am J Clin Nutr* 2000;72:598S-606S.

10. Micheletti A, Rossi R, et al. Zinc status in athletes: relation to diet and exercise. *Sports Med* 2001;31:577-582.

11. Lukaski H. Low dietary zinc decreases erythrocyte carbonic anhydrase activities and impairs cardiorespiratory function in men during exercise. *Am J Clin Nutr* 2005;81:1045-1051.

12. Kelly G. Sports Nutrition: A review of selected nutritional supplements for bodybuilders and strength athletes. *Altern Med Rev* 1997;2:184- 201.

13. Golf S, Bender S, Gruttner J. On the significance of magnesium in extreme physical stress. *Cardiovasc Drugs Ther* 1998;12:197-202.

14. Brilla L, Haley T. Effect of magnesium supplementation on strength training in humans. *J Am Coll Nutr* 1992;11:326-329.

15. Medved I, Brown M, et al. N-acetylcysteine enhances muscle cysteine and glutathione availability and attenuates fatigue during prolonged exercise in endurance-trained individuals. *J Appl Physiol* 2004;97:1477-1485.

16. Medved I, Brown M, Bjorksten A, et al. Effects of intravenous N-acetylcysteine infusion on time to fatigue and potassium regulation during prolonged cycling exercise. *J Appl Physiol* 2004;96:211-217.

17. Sekhar R, Patel S, Guthikonda A, et al. Deficient synthesis of glutathione underlies oxidative stress in aging and can be corrected by dietary cysteine and glycine supplementation. *Am J Clin Nutr* 2011;94:847-853.

18. Starks M, Starks S, et al. The effects of phosphatidylserine on endocrine response to moderate intensity exercise. *J Int Soc Sports Nutr* 2008;5:11.

19. Monteleone P, Bienat L, Tanzillo C, et al. Effects of phosphatidylserine on the neuroendocrine response to physical stress in humans. *Neuroendocrinology* 1990;52:243-248.

20. Kingsley M, Miller M, KIlduff L, et al. Effects of phosphatidylserine on exercise capacity during cycling in

active males. *Med Sci Sports Exerc* 2006;38:64-71.
21. Marquezi M, Roschel H, et al. Effect of aspartate and asparagine supplementation on fatigue determinants in intense exercise. *Int J Sport Nutr Exer Metab* 2003;13:65-75. 33.
22. Lancha A, Recco M, et al. Effect of aspartate, asparagine, and carnitine supplementation in the diet on metabolism of skeletal muscle during a moderate exercise. *Physiol Behav* 1995;57:367-371.
23. Pitkanen H, Mero A, Oja S, et al. Effects of training on the exercise-induced changes in serum amino acids and hormones. *J Strength Cond Res* 2002;16:390-398.
24. Agostini F, Biolo G. Effect of physical activity on glutamine metabolism. *Curr Opin Clin Nutr Metab Care* 2010;13:58-64.
25. Castell L, Newsholme E. The effects of oral glutamine supplementation on athletes after prolonged, exhaustive exercise. *Nutrition* 1997;13:738-742.
26. Rowbottom D, Keast D, Morton A. The emerging role of glutamine as an indicator of exercise stress and overtraining. *Sports Med* 1996;21:80-97.
27. Keast D, Arstein D, Harper W, et al. Depression of plasma glutamine concentration after exercise stress and its possible influence on the immune system. *Med J Aust* 1995;162:15-18.
28. Alf D, Schmidt M, Siebrecht S. Ubiquinol supplementation enhances peak power production in trained athletes: a double-blind, placebo controlled study. *J Int Soc Sport Nutr* 2013;10:24.
29. Diaz-Castro J, Guisado R, Kajarabille N, et al. Coenzyme Q10 supplementation ameliorates inflammatory signaling and oxidative stress associated with strenuous exercise. *Eur J Nutr* 2012;51:791-799.
30. Mizuno K, Tanaka M, Nozaki S, et al. Anti-fatigue effects of coenzyme Q10 during physical fatigue. *Nutrition* 2008;24:293-299.
31. Zembron-Lacny A, Szyszka K, Szygula Z. Effect of cysteine derivatives administration in healthy men exposed to intense resistance exercise by evaluation of pro-antioxidant ratio. *J Phsyiol Sci* 2007;57:343-348.

32. Zembron-Lacny A, Slowinska-Lisowska M, Szyfula Z, et al. Assessment of the antioxidant effectiveness of alpha-lipoic acid in healthy men exposed to muscle-damaging exercise. *J Phsyiol Pharmacol* 2009;60:139-143.
33. Kretzschmar M, Müller D. Aging, training and exercise. A review of effects on plasma glutathione and lipid peroxides. *Sports Med* 1993;15:196-209.
34. Leeuwenburgh C, Leichtweis S, Hollander J, et al. Effect of acute exercise in glutathione deficiency heart. *Mol Cell Biochem* 1996;156:17- 24.
35. Giamberardino M, Dragani L, Valente R, et al. Effects of prolonged L-carnitine administration on delayed muscle pain and CK release after eccentric effort. *Int J Sports Med* 1996;17:320-324.
36. Ho J, Kraemer W, Volek J, et al. L-Carnitine, L-tartrate supplementation favorably affects biochemical markers of recovery from physical exertion in middle-aged men and women. *Metabolism* 2010;59:1190-1199.

Additional references at
http://www.spectracell.com/clinicians/clinical-education-center/online-library-mnt-sports-medicine-abstracts/

Some content adapted from SpectraCell Laboratories, Inc.

Telomeres

Telomeres, the caps at the end of each strand of DNA that protects chromosome, are an essential part of human cells affecting how cells age. Vitamins are needed to keep these healthy. Folate influences telomere length through DNA methylation.[1,2,3] Vitamin B3 (niacin) extends the lifespan of human cells in vitro and slows the telomere attrition rate by reducing reactive oxygen species in mitochondria.[4,5] Vitamins B2, B6, and B12 are crucial for proper DNA methylation.[6,7] Vitamin C protects DNA from oxidation. In vitro studies show it slows age-related telomere shortening in human skin cells.[8,9] Vitamin E enhances DNA repair as well as removal of damaged DNA. It has been shown in vitro to restore telomere length on human cells.[10,11] Vitamin D positively co-occurs with telomere length due to its anti-inflammatory role.[12]

Healthy telomeres need adequate mineral supplementation. Zinc is an important cofactor for DNA repair enzymes and plays a vital role in managing inflammation.[13,14] Copper is a crucial cofactor in the potent antioxidant superoxide dismutase that is known to protect telomeres.[15] Magnesium regulates chromosome separation in cell replication. From research, a magnesium-induced deficiency shortened telomeres in the livers of rats.[16] On the other hand, in vitro supplementation of selenium extended telomere length in liver cells. Selenoproteins protect DNA.[17,18,19,20] Manganese is a required cofactor in superoxide dismutase, and its deficiency decreases telomerase activity.[21] Calcium is a required cofactor to prevent DNA replication errors [22]

Stem cell treatment with N-acetyl cysteine, an amino acid, corrects DNA damage in telomeres.[23] Interference of glutathione, another amino acid, dependent antioxidant defenses accelerates the erosion of telomere.[24,25]

Reference List

1. Fenech M. Nutriomes and nutrient arrays - the key to personalized nutrition for DNA damage prevention and cancer growth control. *Genome Integr* 2010;1:11.
2. Moores CJ, Fenech M, O'Callaghan NJ. Telomere dynamics: the influence of folate and DNA methylation. *Ann NY Acad Sci* 2011;1229:76-88.

3. Paul L, Cattaneo M, D'Angelo A, et al. Telomere Length in Peripheral Blood Mononuclear Cells is Associated with Folate Status in Men. *J Nutr* 2009;139:1273-1278.

4. Kang HT, Lee HI, Hwang ES. Nicotinamide extends replicative lifespan of human cells. *Aging Cell* 2006;5:423-436.

5. Kirkland JB. Niacin and carcinogenesis. *Nutr Cancer* 2003;46:110-118.

6. Das P, Singal R. DNA methylation and cancer. *J Clin Oncol* 2004;22:4632-4642.

7. Bull CF, O'Callaghan NJ, Mayrhofer G, Fenech MF. Telomere Length in Lymphocytes of Older South Australian Men May Be Inversely Associated with Plasma Homocysteine. *Rejuvenation Res* 2009;12:341-349.

8. Serra V, von Zglinicki T, Lorenz M, Saretzki G. Extracellular superoxide dismutase is a major antioxidant in human fibroblasts and slows telomere shortening. *J Biol Chem* 2003;278:6824-6830.

9. Martin H, Uring-Lambert B, Adrian M, et al. Effects of long-term dietary intake of magnesium on oxidative stress, apoptosis and ageing in rat liver. *Magnes Res* 2008;21:124-130.

10. Liu Q, Wang H, Hu D, et al. Effects of trace elements on the telomere lengths of hepatocytes L-02 and hepatoma cells SMMC-7721. *Biol Trace Elem Res* 2004;100:215-227.

11. McCann JC, Ames BN. Adaptive dysfunction of selenoproteins from the perspective of the triage theory: why modest selenium deficiency may increase risk of diseases of aging. *FASEB J* 2011;25:1793-1814.

12. Jackson M, Combs GF Jr. Selenium and anticarcinogenesis: underlying mechanisms. *Curr Opin Clin Nutr Metab Care* 2008;11:718-726.

13. Sharif R, Thomas P, Zalewski P, Fenech M. The role of zinc in genomic stability. *Mutat Res* 2011; Epub ahead of print.

14. Cipriano C, Tesei S, Malavolta M, et al. Accumulation of cells with short telomeres is associated with impaired zinc homeostasis and inflammation in old hypertensive participants. *J Gerontol A Biol Sci Med Sci* 2009;64:745-751.

15. Serra V, von Zglinicki T, Lorenz M, Saretzki G. Extracellular superoxide dismutase is a major antioxidant in

---

human fibroblasts and slows telomere shortening. *J Biol Chem* 2003;278:6824-6830.

16. Martin H, Uring-Lambert B, Adrian M, et al. Effects of long-term dietary intake of magnesium on oxidative stress, apoptosis and ageing in rat liver. *Magnes Res*2008;21:124-130.

17. Liu Q, Wang H, Hu D, et al. Effects of trace elements on the telomere lengths of hepatocytes L-02 and hepatoma cells SMMC-7721. *Biol Trace Elem Res* 2004;100:215-227.

18. McCann JC, Ames BN. Adaptive dysfunction of selenoproteins from the perspective of the triage theory: why modest selenium deficiency may increase risk of diseases of aging. *FASEB J* 2011;25:1793-1814.

19. Jackson M, Combs GF Jr. Selenium and anticarcinogenesis: underlying mechanisms. *Curr Opin Clin Nutr Metab Care* 2008;11:718-726.

20. Schnabel R, Lubos E, Messow C, et al. Selenium supplementation improves antioxidant capacity in vitro and in vivo in patients with coronary artery disease The Selenium Therapy in Coronary Artery Disease Patients (SETCAP) Study. *Am Heart J* 2008;156:1201.e1-1211.

21. Makino N, Maeda T, Oyama J, et al. Antioxidant therapy attenuates myocardial telomerase activity reduction in superoxide dismutase-deficient mice. *J Mol Cell Cardiol* 2011;50:670-677.

22. Chandra S. Subcellular imaging of RNA distribution and DNA replication in single mammalian cells with SIMS: the localization of heat shock induced RNA in relation to the distribution of intranuclear bound calcium. *J Microsc* 2008;232:27-35.

23. Gu BW, Fan JM, Bessler M, Mason PJ. Accelerated hematopoietic stem cell aging in aging mouse model of dyskeratosis congenita responds to antioxidant treatment. *Aging Cell* 2011;10:338-348.

24. Kurz D, Decary S, Hong Y, et al. Chronic oxidative stress compromises telomere integrity and accelerates the onset of senescence in human endothelial cells. *J Cell Sci* 2004;117:2417-2426.

25. Watfa G, Dragonas C, Brosche T, et al. Study of telomere length and different markers of oxidative stress in patients

---

with Parkinson's disease. *J Nutr Health Aging* 2011;15:277-281.

Some content adapted from SpectraCell Laboratories, Inc.

Testosterone

Adequate levels of testosterone are necessary for good health for men and women (see testosterone chapter in *13 Secrets of Optimal Aging)*. Its production is related to the intake of several micronutrients. There is an important interplay between folate and testosterone. A folate deficiency decreases circulating testosterone, and evidence suggests that testosterone may regulate folate metabolism.[1,2,3] Vitamin B6 regulates sex hormones and reduces prolactin that stimulates the hypothalamus to increase testosterone. It is also a cofactor for dopamine synthesis that influences testosterone levels.[4,5,6,7] Supplementation with Vitamin D, a hormone that regulates the synthesis of testosterone, can significantly increase total, free, and bioactive testosterone levels.[8,9,10,11,12] A Vitamin K deficiency decreases testosterone production because the rate-limiting enzyme for testosterone synthesis (Cyp11a) is Vitamin K dependent.[13,14,15] Long term administration of some forms of Vitamin E may reduce testosterone levels.[16,17] Vitamin C studies suggest it protects the prostate and testicles from tumors.[18,19,20]

Minerals also interact with testosterone. Magnesium makes testosterone more biologically active in the body and raises free and total testosterone levels in men.[21-23] A zinc deficiency lowers testosterone levels because it inhibits prolactin secretion (a testosterone inhibiting hormone). Supplementation with zinc increases testosterone, depending on baseline levels.[24-27] The amino acid carnitine boosts dopamine and may prevent testosterone decline after intense physical stress.[28-31]

Reference List

1. Wallock-Montelius L, Villanueva J, Chapin R et al. Chronic ethanol perturbs testicular folate metabolism ciency reduces sex hormone levels in the Yucatan micropig. *Biol Reprod* 2007;76:455-465.
2. Rovinetti C, Bovina C, Tolomeli B, et al. Effects of testosterone on the metabolism of folate coenzymes in the rat. *Biochem J* 1972;126:291-294.
3. Dudkowska M, Befer S, Jawosrki T, et al. Effects of testosterone on the metabolism of folate coenzymes in the rat. *Biochem J* 1972;126:291-294.

4. Allgood V, Cidlowski J. Vitamin B6 modulates transcriptional activation by multiple members of the steroid hormone receptor superfamily. *J Biol Chem* 1992;25:3819-3824.

5. Ren S, Melmed S, Pyridoxal phosphate inhibits pituitary cell proliferation and hormone secretion. *Endocrinology* 2006;147:3936-3942.

6. Hoffman A, Melmed S, Schlechte J. Patient guide to hyperprolactinemia diagnosis and treatment. *J Clin Endocrinol Metab* 2011;96:35A-6A.

7. Guilarte T, Wagner H, Frost J. Effects of perinatal Vitamin B6 deficiency on dopaminergic neurochemistry. *J Neurochem* 1987;48:432-439.

8. Pilz S, Frisch S, koertke H, et al. Effect of vitamin D supplementation on testosterone levels in men. *Hormone Metab Res* 2011;43:223-225.

9. Bloomberg M. Vitamin D metabolism, sex hormones and male reproductive function. *Reproduction* 2012;144:135-152.

10. Nimptsch K, Platz E, Willett W, et al. Association between plasma 25-OH Vitamin D and testosterone levels in men. *Clin Edocrinol* 2012;166:77-85.

11. Lee D, Tajar A, Pye S, et al. Association of hypogonadism with Vitamin D status: the European Male Ageing Study. *Eur J Endocrinol* 2012;166:77-85.

12. Wehr E, Pilz S, Boehm B, et al. Association of Vitamin D status with serum androgen levels in men. *Clin Endocrinol* 2010;73:243-248.

13. Shirikawa H, Ohsaki y, Minegishi T, et al. Viatmin K deficiency reduces testosterone production in the testis through down-regulation of the Cyp11a a cholesterol side chain cleavage enzyme in rats. *Biochim Biophys Acta* 2006; 1760:1482-1488.

14. Takumi N, Shirakawa H Ohsaki Y et al. Dietary Vitamin K alleviates the reduction in testosterone production induced by lipopolysaccharide administration in rat testis. *Food Funct* 2011;2:406-411.

15. Ito A, Shirakawa H, Takumi N, et al. Menaquione-4 enhances testosterone production in rats and testisderived tumor cells. *Lipids Health Dis* 2011;10:158.

16. Hartman T, Dorgan J, Woodson K, et al. Effects of long-term

alpha-tocopherol supplementation on serum hormones in older men. *Prostate* 2001;46:33-38.

17. Hartman T, Dorgran K, Virtamo J, et al. Association between serum alpha-tocopherol and serum androgens and estrogens in older men. *Nutr Cancer* 1999;35:10-15.

18. Li S, Ryu J, Park S, et al. Vitamin C supplementation prevents testosterone-induced hyperplasia of rat prostate by dow-regulating HIF-1alpha. *J Nutr Biochem* 2010;21:801-808.

19. Ripple M, Henry W, Rago R, et al. Prooxidant-antioxidant shift induced by androgen treatment of human prostate carcinoma cells. *J Natl Cancer Inst* 1997;89:40-48.

20. Das U, Mallick M, Debnath J, et al. Protective effect of ascorbic acid on cyclophosphamide-induced testicular gametogenic and androgenic disorders in male rats. *Asi J Androl* 2002;4:201-207.

21. Maggio M, Ceda G, Lauretani F, et al. Effects of magnesium and anabolic hormones in older men. *Int J Androl* 2011;34:e594-600.

22. Cinar V, Polat Y, Baltaci A, et al. Effects of magnesium supplementation on testosterone levels of athletes and sedentary subjects at rest and exhaustion. *Biol Trace Elem Res* 2011;140:18-23.

23. Excoffon L, Guillaume Y, Woronof-Lemsi M, et al. Magnesium effect on testosterone-SHBG association studied by a novel molecular chromatography approach. *J Pharm Biomed Anal* 2009:49:175-180.

24. Prasad A, Mantzoros C, Beck F, et al. Zinc status and serum testosterone levels of healthy adults. *Nutrition* 1996;12:344-348.

25. Netter A, Hartoma R, Nahoul K. Effect of zinc administration on plasma testosterone, dihydrostestosterone, and sperm count. *Arch Androl* 1981;7:69-73.

26. Jalali GR, Roozbeh J, Mohammadzadeh A, et al. Impact of oral zinc therapy on the level of sex hormones in male patients on hemodialysis. *Ren Fail* 2010;32:417-419.

27. Costello L, Liu Y, Zou J, et al. Evidence for a zinc uptake transporter in human prostate cancer cells which is regulated by prolactin and testosterone. *J Biol Chem* 1999;274:17499-17504.

28. Maggio M, Ceda G, Lauretani F, et al. Effects of magnesium and anabolic hormones in older men. *Int J Androl* 2011;34:e594-600.
29. Cinar V, Polat Y, Baltaci A, et al. Effects of magnesium supplementation on testosterone levels of athletes and sedentary subjects at rest and exhaustion. *Biol Trace Elem Res* 2011;140:18-23.
30. Excoffon L, Guillaume Y, Woronof-Lemsi M, et al. Magnesium effect on testosterone-SHBG association studied by a novel molecular chromatography approach. *J Pharm Biomed Anal* 2009:49:175-180.
31. Prasad A, Mantzoros C, Beck F, et al. Zinc status and serum testosterone levels of healthy adults. *Nutrition* 1996;12:344-348.

Some content adapted from SpectraCell Laboratories, Inc.

Weight Management (See Obesity)

With the increase of obesity and its related health problems, many people are interested in better managing their weight. Vitamin supplementation is necessary to achieve optimum results. Biotin boosts metabolism by improving glycemic control by stabilizing blood sugar and lowering insulin, a hormone that promotes fat formation.[1-3] Vitamin B5 (pantothenic acid) lowers body weight by activating lipoprotein lipase, an enzyme that burns fat cells. One study linked B5 supplementation to less hunger when dieting.[4,5] Inositol supplementation may increase levels of adiponectin, a protein involved in regulating glucose levels and fatty acid breakdown.[6]

Treatment with B3 (niacin) increases adiponectin, a weight-loss hormone secreted by fat cells. Niacin-bound chromium supplements helped reduced body weight in clinical studies.[7-9] Vitamin A promotes expression of genes that reduce a person's tendency to store food as fat and reduces the size of fat cells.[10-12] Vitamin E inhibits pre-fat cells from changing into mature fat cells, thereby reducing body fat.[12-14] A Vitamin D deficiency is strongly linked to poor metabolism of carbohydrates. Genes that are regulated by Vitamin D may alter the way fat cells form in some people.[15-17] Poor Vitamin K status co-occurs with excess fat tissue, and Vitamin K helps to metabolize sugars.[18,19]

Adequate mineral intake is needed for ideal weight management. Calcium inhibits the formation of fat cells and also helps oxidize (burn) fat cells.[12,16,20] Chromium makes the body more sensitive to insulin, helping to decrease body fat and increase lean muscle.[21-26] Low magnesium in cells impairs a person's ability to use glucose for fuel, instead storing it as fat. Correcting a magnesium deficiency stimulates metabolism by increasing insulin sensitivity. Magnesium may also inhibit fat absorption.[27-29] A zinc deficiency reduces leptin, a beneficial hormone that regulates appetite, which is reversed by bringing zinc up to optimum levels.[12,30]

Amino acids are essential. Asparagine, which increases insulin sensitivity, helps the body store energy in muscle instead of storing it as body fat.[31,32] Supplementaion with cysteine reduced body fat in obese patients.[33] Carnitine carries fatty acids into the cell so they can be burned for fuel, and, therefore, reduce visceral adiposity (belly fat).[34,35] Lipoic acid enhances glucose uptake into

This enhancement helps a person burn carbohydrates more efficiently.[36-38]Glutamine reduces fat mass by increasing glucose uptake into muscle.[39,40]

Reference List

1. Larrieta E, de la Vega-Monroy M, Vital P, et al. Effects of biotin deficiency on pancreatic islet morphology, insulin sensitivity and glucose homeostasis. *J Nutr Biochem* 2012;4:392-399.
2. Albarracin C, Fuqua B, Evans J, et al. Chromium picolinate and biotin combination improves glucose metabolism in treated, uncontrolled overweight to obese patients with type 2 diabetes. *Diabetes Metab Res* 2008;1:41-51.
3. Monograph on Biotin. *Altern Med Rev* 2007;12:73-78.
4. Naruta E, Buko V. Hypolipidemic effect of pantothenic acid derivatives in mice with hypothalamic obesity induced by aurothioglucose. *Exp Toxicol Pathol* 2001;5:393-398.
5. Leung L. Pantothenic acid as a weight-reducing agent: fasting without hunger, weakness and ketosis. *Med Hypotheses* 1995;5:403-405.
6. Corrado F, D'anna R, Di Vieste G, et al. The effect of myoinositol supplementation on insulin resistance in patients with gestational diabetes. *Diabet Med* 2011;8:972-975.
7. Westpahl S, Borucki K, Taneva E, et al. Adipokines and treatment with niacin. *Metabolism* 2006;10:1283-1285.
8. Rink C, Roy S, Khanna S, et al. Transcriptome of the subcutaneous adipose tissue in response to oral supplementation of type 2 Leprdb obese diabetic mice with niacin-bound chromium. *Physiol Genomics* 2006;3:370-379.
9. Preuss H, Bagchi D, Bagchi M, et al. Effects of a natural extract of (-)-hydroxycitric acid (HCA-SX) and a combination of HCA-SX plus niacin-bound chromium and Gymnema sylvestre extract on weight loss. *Diabetes Obes Metab* 2004;3:171-180.
10. Kameji H, Mochizuki K, Myoshi N et al. β-Carotene accumulation in 3T3-L1 adipocytes inhibits the elevation of reactive oxygen species and the suppression of genes related to insulin sensitivity induced by tumor necrosis factor-α. *Nutrition* 2010;11-12:1151-1156.

_____

11. Ribot J, Felipe F, Bonet M, el al. Changes in adiposity in response to vitamin A status correlate with changes of PPAR gamma 2 expression. *Obes Res* 2001;9:500-509.

12. Garcia O, Long K, Rosado J. Impact of micronutrient deficiencies on obesity. *Nutr Rev* 2009;10:559-572.

13. Ohrvall M, Tengblad S, Vessby B. Lower tocopherol serum levels in subjects with abdominal adiposity. *J Intern Med* 1993;234:53-60.

14. Uto-Kondo H, Ohmori R, Kiyose C, et al. Tocotrienol Suppresses Adipocyte Differentiation and Akt Phosphorylation in 3T3-L1 Preadipocytes. *J Nutr* 2009;1:51-57.

15. Bailey R, Cooper J, Zeitels K, et al. Association of the vitamin D metabolism gene CYP27B1 with type I diabetes. *Diabetes* 2007;10:2616-2621.

16. Bailey R, Cooper J, Zeitels K, et al. Association of the vitamin D metabolism gene CYP27B1 with type I diabetes. *Diabetes* 2007;10:2616-2621.

17. Ochs-Balcom H, Chennamaneni R, Millen A, et al. Vitamin D receptor genepolymorphisms are associated with adiposity phenotypes. *Am J Clin Nutr* 2011;1:5-10.

18. Yoshida M, Jacques P, Meigs J, et al. Effect of vitamin K supplementation on insulin resistance in older men and women. *Diabetes Care* 2008;11:2092-2096.

19. Shea M, Booth S, Gundberg C. et al. Adulthood obesity is positively associated with adipose tissue concentrations of vitamin K and inversely associated with circulating indicators of vitamin K status in men and women. *J Nutr* 2010;5:1029-1034.

20. Zernal M. Role of calcium and dairy products in energy partitioning and weight management. *Am J Clin Nutr* 2004;79(Suppl):S907-S912.

21. Kim C, Kim B, Park K, et al. Effects of short-term chromium supplementation on insulin sensitivity and body composition in overweight children: randomized, double-blind, placebo-controlled study. *J Nutr Biochem* 2011;11:1030-1034.

22. Lau F, Bagchi M, Sen C, et al. Nutrigenomic basis of beneficial effects of chromium(III) on obesity and diabetes. *Mol Cell Biochem* 2008;1-2:1-10.

23. Cefalu W, Rood J, Pinsonat P, et al. Characterization of the

metabolic and physiologic response to chromium supplementation in subjects with type 2 diabetes mellitus. *Metabolism* 2010;5:755-762.

24. Rink C, Roy S, Khanna S, et al. Transcriptome of the subcutaneous adipose tissue in response to oral supplementation of type 2 Leprdb obese diabetic mice with niacin-bound chromium. *Physiol Genomics* 2006;3:370-379.

25. Preuss H, Bagchi D, Bagchi M, et al. Effects of a natural extract of (-)-hydroxycitric acid (HCA-SX) and a combination of HCA-SX plus niacin-bound chromium and Gymnema sylvestre extract on weight loss. *Diabetes Obes Metab* 2004;3:171-180.

26. Albarracin C, Fuqua B, Evans J, et al. Chromium picolinate and biotin combination improves glucose metabolism in treated, uncontrolled overweight to obese patients with type 2 diabetes. *Diabetes Metab Res* 2008;1:41-51.

27. Takaya J, Higashino H, KobayashiY. Intracellular magnesium and insulin resistance.*Magnes Res* 2004;2:126-36.

28. Kishimoto Y, Tani M, Uto-Kondo H, et al. Effects of magnesium on postprandial serum lipid responses in healthy human subjects. *Br J Nutr* 2010;4:469-472.

29. Lima M, Cruz T, Rodrigues L, et al. Serum and intracellular magnesium deficiency in patients with metabolic syndrome--evidences for its relation to insulin resistance. *Diabetes Res Clin Pract* 2009;2:257-262.

30. Jansen J, et al. Zinc and diabetes--clinical links and molecular mechanisms. *J Nutr Biochem* 2009;6:399-417.

31. Lancha A, Poortmans J, Pereira L. The effect of 5 days of aspartate and asparagine supplementation on glucose transport activity in rat muscle. *Cell Biochem Funct* 2009;8:552-557.

32. Marquezi M, Roschel H, et al. Effect of aspartate and asparagine supplementation on fatigue determinants in intense exercise. *Int J Sport Nutr Exer Metab* 2003;13:65-75.

33. Hildebrandt W, Hamman A, Krakowsi-Roosen H, et al. Effect of thiol antioxidant on body fat and insulin reactivity. *J Mol Med* 2004;5:336-344.

34. Bernard A, Rigault C, Mazue F, et al. L-carnitine supplementation and physical exercise restore age-associated

decline in some mitochondrial functions in the rat. *J Gerontol A Biol Sci Med Sci* 2008;10:1027-1033.

35. Galloway S, Craig T, Cleland S. Effects of oral L-carnitine supplementation on insulin sensitivity indices in response to glucose feeding in lean and overweight/obese males. *Amino Acids* 2011;2:507-515.

36. Teachey M, Taylor Z, Maier T, et al. Interactions of conjugated linoleic acid and lipoic acid on insulin action in the obese Zucker rat. *Metabolism* 2003;9:1167-1174.

37. Zhang Y, Han P, Wu N, et al. Amelioration of Lipid Abnormalities by α-Lipoic acid Through Antioxidative and Anti- Inflammatory Effects. *Obesity* 2011;8:1647-1653.

38. Ansar H, Mazloom Z, Kazemi F et al. Effect of alpha-lipoic acid on blood glucose, insulin resistance and glutathione peroxidase of type 2 diabetic patients. *Saudi Med J* 2011;6:584-588.

39. Greenfield J, Farooqi I, Keogh J, et al. Oral glutamine increases circulating glucagon-like peptide 1, glucagon, and insulin concentrations in lean, obese, and type 2 diabetic subjects. *Am J Clin Nutr* 2009;1:106-113.

40. Prada P, Hirabara S, de Souza C, et al. L-glutamine supplementation induces insulin resistance in adipose tissue and improves insulin signalling in liver and muscle of rats with diet-induced obesity. *Diabetologia* 2007;9:1949-59.

Some content adapted from SpectraCell Laboratories, Inc.

Women's Health

There are several health conditions that tend to occur more frequently in women than in men: osteoporosis, PMS, menopause, and breast cancer, for example. Vitamin deficiencies are associated with chronic disease processes and the overall condition of a woman's health. For osteoporosis, Vitamin K is a major factor in building bone proteins.[1,2] Vitamin D can lessen premenstrual headaches[3,4] and can decrease bacterial infections during pregnancy.[5,6] Folic acid and B Vitamin supplementation in women can help blood vessels remain pliable and clear while improving a woman's lipid profile after menopause.[7] Vitamin A has been shown to reduce DNA damage in cancerous tissue and inhibit hormonal toxicities that can initiate cancerous cells.[8,9] Vitamin A and B2 can alleviate pregnancy anemia.[10,11] Folic acid, biotin, and B Vitamins may help in the reduction of birth defects.[12,13]

Women need sufficient minerals to maintain good health. Calcium in conjunction with Vitamins D, K, and C helps to prevent osteoporosis.[14,15] This combination also helps to alleviate symptoms of PMS (premenstrual syndrome). Vitamin D and calcium are also necessary to lower the risk of breast cancer.[16,17] In some women, high estrogen levels during menopause are associated with low magnesium level, which then affects blood pressure.[18] In clinical studies, zinc has reduced and sometimes eliminated menstrual cramping.[19] Also, a zinc deficiency can negatively affect bone integrity.[20,21] Calcium and magnesium plus Vitamin B6 supplementation can reduce the anxiety that women often feel during PMS.[22] Trace elements can reduce pregnancy-induced hypertension.[23-24]

Finally, the amino acid carnitine can improve bone mineral density.[25,26] Coenzyme Q10 and selenium reduce the risk of pre-eclampsia during pregnancy.[28,29]

Reference List

1. Villa JK, Diaz MA, Pizziolo VR, Martino HS. Effect of vitamin K in bone metabolism and vascular calcification: a review of mechanisms of action and evidences. *Crit Rev Food Sci Nutr.* 2016 Jul 20:0. [Epub ahead of print] PMID: 27437760.

2. Maresz K. Proper Calcium Use: Vitamin K2 as a Promoter of Bone and Cardiovascular Health. Maresz K. *Integr Med* (Encinitas). 2015 Feb;14(1):34-9. Review. PMID: 26770129.

3. Obeidat BA, Alchalabi HA, Abdul-Razzak KK, Al-Farras MI.Premenstrual symptoms in dysmenorrheic college students: prevalence and relation to vitamin Dand parathyroid hormone levels. *Int J Environ Res Public Health.* 2012 Nov 16;9(11):4210-22. doi: 10.3390/ijerph9114210. PMID: 23202842.

4. Thys-Jacobs S. Vitamin D and calcium in menstrual migraine. *Headache.* 1994 Oct;34(9):544-6. PMID: 8002332.

5. Skowrońska-Jóźwiak E, Lebiedzińska K, Smyczyńska J, et al.Effects of maternal vitamin D status on pregnancy outcomes, health of pregnant women and their offspring. *Neuro Endocrinol Lett.* 2014;35(5):367-72. PMID: 25275261.

6. Hensel KJ, Randis TM, Gelber SE, Ratner AJ. Pregnancy-specific association of vitamin D deficiency and bacterial vaginosis. *Am J Obstet Gynecol.* 2011 Jan;204(1):41.e1-9. doi: 10.1016/j.ajog.2010.08.013. Epub 2010 Oct 8. PMID: 20887971.

7. Paradisi G, Cucinelli F, Mele MC, Barini A, Lanzone A, Caruso A. Endothelial function in post-menopausal women: effect of folic acid supplementation. *Hum Reprod.* 2004 Apr;19(4):1031-5. Epub 2004 Mar 11. PMID: 15016776.

8. Bakker MF, Peeters PH, Klaasen VM, et al. Plasma carotenoids, vitamin C, tocopherols, and retinol and the risk of breast cancer in the European Prospective Investigation into Cancer and Nutrition cohort. *Am J Clin Nutr.* 2016 Feb;103(2):454-64. doi: 10.3945/ajcn.114.101659. Epub 2016 Jan 20. PMID: 26791185.

9. Maggio M, de Vita F, Lauretani F, et al. Relationship between Carotenoids, Retinol, and Estradiol Levels in Older Women. *Nutrients.* 2015 Aug 5;7(8):6506-19. doi: 10.3390/nu7085296. PMID: 26251919.

10. Yang f, Ma AG, Zhang XZ, Jiang DC. Status of vitamin A,

vitamin B2, iron and an-oxidative activity in anemic pregnant women in China]. *Wei Sheng Yan Jiu.* 2006 May;35(3):320-2. Chinese. PMID: .16921759

11. Suprapto B, Widardo, Suhanantyo. Effect of low-dosage vitamin A and riboflavin on iron-folate supplementation in anaemic pregnant women. *Asia Pac J Clin Nutr.* 2002;11(4):263-7. PMID: 12495257.

12. Arth A, Kancherla V, Pachón H, et al. A 2015 global update on folic acid-preventable spina bifida and anencephaly. *Birth Defects Res A Clin Mol Teratol.* 2016 Jul;106(7):520-9. doi: 10.1002/bdra.23529. PMID: 27418029.

13. Gannavarapu S, Prasad C, DiRaimo J, et al. Biotinidase deficiency: Spectrum of molecular, enzymatic and clinical information from newborn screening Ontario, Canada (2007-2014). *Mol Genet Metab.* 2015 Nov;116(3):146-51. doi: 10.1016/j.ymgme.2015.08.010. Epub 2015 Aug 31. PMID: 26361991.

14. Nieves JW. Skeletal effects of nutrients and nutraceuticals, beyond calcium and vitamin D. Nieves JW. *Osteoporos Int.* 2013 Mar;24(3):771-86. doi: 10.1007/s00198-012-2214-4. Epub 2012 Nov 14. Review. PMID: 23152094.

15. Ahmadieh H, Arabi A. Vitamins and bone health: beyond calcium and vitamin D. *Nutr Rev.* 2011 Oct;69(10):584-98. doi: 10.1111/j.1753-4887.2011.00372.x. Review. PMID: 21967159.

16. Anderson LN, Cotterchio M, Vieth R, Knight JA. Vitamin D and calcium intakes and breast cancer risk in pre- and postmenopausal women. *Am J Clin Nutr.* 2010 Jun;91(6):1699-707. doi: 10.3945/ajcn.2009.28869. Epub 2010 Apr 14. PMID: 20392891.

17. McCullough ML, Rodriguez C, Diver WR, et al. Dairy, calcium, and vitamin D intake and postmenopausal breast cancer risk in the Cancer Prevention Study II Nutrition Cohort. *Cancer Epidemiol Biomarkers Prev.* 2005 Dec;14(12):2898-904. PMID: 16365007.

18. Nielsen FH, Milne DB, Klevay LM, Gallagher S, Johnson L. Dietary magnesium deficiency induces heart rhythm changes, impairs glucose tolerance, and decreases serum

cholesterol in post-menopausal women. *J Am Coll Nutr.* 2007 Apr;26(2):121-32. PMID: 17536123.

19. Eby GA. Zinc treatment prevents dysmenorrhea. *Med Hypotheses.* 2007;69(2):297-301. Epub 2007 Feb 7.

20. Mahdavi-Roshan M, Ebrahimi M, Ebrahimi A. Copper, magnesium, zinc and calcium status in osteopenic and osteoporotic post-menopausal women. *Clin Cases Miner Bone Metab.* 2015 Jan-Apr;12(1):18-21. doi:10.11138/ccmbm/2015.12.1.018. Review. PMID: 26136790.

21. Zheng J, Mao X, Ling J, He Q, Quan J. Low serum levels of zinc, copper, and iron as risk factors for osteoporosis: a meta-analysis. *Biol Trace Elem Res.* 2014 Jul;160(1):15-23. doi: 10.1007/s12011-014-0031-7. Epub 2014 Jun 8. Review. PMID: 24908111.

22. De Souza MC, Walker AF, Robinson PA, Bolland K. Synergistic effect of a daily supplement for 1 month of 200 mg magnesium plus 50 mg vitamin B6for the relief of anxiety-related premenstrual symptoms: a randomized, double-blind, crossover study. *J Womens Health Gend Based Med.* 2000 Mar;9(2):131-9. PMID: 10746516.

23. Wen SW, Guo Y, Rodger M, et al. Folic Acid Supplementation in Pregnancy and the Risk of Pre-Eclampsia-A Cohort Study. *PLoS One.* 2016 Feb 22;11(2):e0149818. doi: 10.1371/journal.pone.0149818. eCollection 2016. PMID: 26901463.

24. Ma Y, Shen X, Zhang D. The Relationship between Serum Zinc Level and Preeclampsia: A Meta-Analysis. *Nutrients.* 2015 Sep 15;7(9):7806-20. doi: 10.3390/nu7095366. Review. PMID: 26389947.

25. Aydin A, Halici Z, Albayrak A, et al. Treatment with Carnitine Enhances Bone Fracture Healing under Osteoporotic and/or Inflammatory Conditions. *Basic Clin Pharmacol Toxicol.* 2015 Sep;117(3):173-9. doi: 10.1111/bcpt.12384. Epub 2015 Feb 19. PMID: 25625309.

26. Hooshmand S, Balakrishnan A, Clark RM, Owen KQ, Koo SI, Arjmandi BH. Dietary l-carnitine supplementation improves bone mineral density by suppressing bone turnover in aged ovariectomized rats. *Phytomedicine.* 2008

Aug;15(8):595-601. doi: 10.1016/j.phymed.2008.02.026. Epub 2008 Jun 9. PMID: 18539446.
27. Hooshmand S, Balakrishnan A, Clark RM, Owen KQ, Koo SI, Arjmandi BH. Coenzyme Q10 supplementation during pregnancy reduces the risk of pre-eclampsia. *Int J Gynaecol Obstet.* 2009 Apr;105(1):43-5. doi: 10.1016/j.ijgo.2008.11.033. Epub 2009 Jan 19. PMID: 19154996.
28. Farzin L, Sajadi F. Comparison of serum trace element levels in patients with or without pre-eclampsia. *J Res Med Sci.* 2012 Oct;17(10):938-41. PMID: 23825993.

Some content adapted from SpectraCell Laboratories, Inc.

Last chapter: Personalized Nutrition Just for You

A common problem I see in my practice is that many patients come in with a long list of supplements or nutraceutical formulas they are already taking—sometimes 20+ bottles. Many times there is a duplication of certain nutrients, such as B Vitamins, Vitamin C, or Vitamin D, in multiple formulations. Sometimes they're taking individual bottles of the B Vitamins such as biotin, folate, or B12 in addition to a B complex formula. At the other end of the spectrum are those not taking any nutritional supplements or cheap synthetic one-a-day multivitamin/mineral products. Recently, the New York Attorney General went to a few discount stores and pulled multiple products off the shelves from multiple different retail chains and, after testing, found 75% of the products did not contain the ingredients listed on the bottle. This is outrageous. Consumers beware.

Another common problem that occurs after testing with satisfying a deficiency is that each individual nutrient has to be ordered separately to get the required level of repletion. Intracellular nutritional deficiencies can take 6-8 months for total body repletion. In the past I have tried to consolidate the number of different bottles of supplements the patient is taking to help reduce redundancy and costs and improved compliance. Even though I used multiple different product lines there was always an overlapping redundancy of certain nutrients. After micronutrient testing was conducted, I often had to special order 4-6 specific nutrients at the therapeutic dosage needed. This usually meant the patient was now taking 4-6 nutritional supplements each in their own bottle.

This is all in the past. Now I have a better and more efficient way to dose patients. I had been looking for years for a company that would make customized nutraceutical from scratch for patients. This is a more efficient and cost effective way to dose nutraceutical than combining multiple different formulas. Making a customized blend of nutraceuticals specific to an individual eliminates the multiple bottles and redundancy while reducing the overall costs to the patient. Eighty to ninety percent of these ingredients can now be custom blended for an individual and dispenses in personalized blister packs for AM and PM dosing.

The dosing is recommended for those times that will allow best absorption and utilization. The patient no longer needs to

---

remember if they are to take a specific nutrient in the morning or evening. It is already divided up appropriately for them. However, you do still have to remember to take them at breakfast and dinner. It has been my experience that this reduces the cost of expenditure on nutraceutical supplementation from anywhere from one quarter to one third of what the patient was paying before. There are instances when an individual will still need separate dosing for specific conditions, but this need has been lessened now, using this new process.

The baseline for supplementation can be accomplished by using a questionnaire that includes genetic, environmental exposures, family history, personal history, age, sex, ethnicity, current prescription and over-the counter medications, conditions suffering from, and current lifestyle of eating, drinking, sleeping, exercise, and stress levels. Information from thyroid, sex hormone, genetics, micronutrients testing, and the like can be added as well. The questionnaire uses a logrithym containing some 5, 470 different variables and is constantly being updated as new data becomes available. There are a potential 1.7 million different outcomes depending upon what information is entered. The logrithym uses a database off thousands of referenced studies on the nutritional relationship to medications, genetics, family history, age, sex, ethnicity, over 300 different conditions, and more.

This process is the only patented process I am aware of that automatically makes recommendations to replenish nutrients that become depleted from prescription and over-the-counter medications. In addition, the software eliminates any ingredients that are contra-indicated. The doctor might forget, but the computer will not. This profile provides a baseline of maintenance doses of multiple nutrients. Increased dosages of nutrients can be added to, if needed, to achieve more therapeutic levels as indicated from the micronutrient testing. These increased levels can be added at a fraction of the cost that the consumer would pay elsewhere.

Since using this in my practice, I have been able to reduce the inventory of many products and pass on saving to my patients without sacrificing any quality. I highly recommend this protocol to other doctors and consumers who want to stay healthy. Go to https://idlife.com/assessment?sponsor_id=1222770&Experience= to take the assessment for yourself. Then you can go to my website drkellymiller.com to request a micronutrient test kit to make an appointment for fine-tuning your personalized recommendations.

Final Thoughts

Micronutrient testing is essential for optimal long-term health. Many of my patients were spending hundreds of dollars each month on supplements without knowing definitively what they needed, and they were still missing micronutrients that were vital to their health. Determining your own individual micronutrient needs will save you time, money, and loss of productivity as well as improve the quality of your life. If you have a significant disease or illness, it is essential to determine if there are nutritional deficiencies contributing to that condition. It could be the difference between having a higher quality of life or even life vs. death. Minimally, properly assessing your own individual micronutrient needs can help you stay healthier and less susceptible to illness because your detoxification, anti-oxidation, and immune system is working optimally.

This book and those to follow reveal the significance of the eight variables to our health: genetic variances, environmental toxins, what we eat, what we drink, how we exercise, how we rest, what we breathe, and what we think. What we think is by far the most important because it determines our beliefs, behavior, and lifestyle. It can even influence gene expression as you will learn in the forthcoming book *How Genetic Testing Can Change/Save Your Life.*

For more information visit our website at www.drkellymiller.com. Micronutrient test kits are available on the website.

The next book in the Health Restoration series is named *Invisible Killers! How to Proactively Protect Yourself from Environmental Toxins.* Coming soon!

Cosmopolitan Article

I found this article while doing research on the book called *Saving Our Brains: Causes, Prevention and Treatment of Dementia and Alzheimer's Disease* (pending publication) that I co-authored with one of my great mentors, Dr. Paul Ling Tai. I find it very relative to the need for micronutrient testing. Please note this article is from 1936.

"Modern Miracle Men" – Relating To Proper Food Mineral Balances by Dr. Charles Northen, Reprinted From Cosmopolitan, June 1936

Presented by Mr. Fletcher June 1 1936 and Ordered to be Printed by the United States Government Printing Office Washington: 1936 During the 74th Congress, Second Session, Document No. 264

This is the Unabridged Version of this document.

MODERN MIRACLE MEN

Dr. Charles Northen, Who Builds Health From The Ground Up

This quiet, unballyhooed pioneer and genius in the field of nutrition demonstrates that countless human ills stem from the fact that impoverished soil of America no longer provides plant foods with the mineral elements essential to human nourishment and health! To overcome this alarming condition, he doctors sick soils and, by seeming miracles, raises truly healthy and health-giving fruits and vegetables.

(By Rex Beach)

Do you know that most of us today are suffering from certain dangerous diet deficiencies which cannot be remedied until the depleted soils from which our foods come are brought into proper mineral balance?

The alarming fact is that foods — fruit and vegetables and grains — now being raised on millions of acres of land no longer contain enough of certain needed minerals, are starving us — no matter how much of them we eat!

This talk about minerals is novel and quite startling. In fact, a realization of the importance of minerals in food is so new that the textbooks on nutritional dietetics contain very little about it. Nevertheless it is something that concerns all of us, and the further we delve into it the more startling it becomes.

179

You'd think, wouldn't you, that a carrot is a carrot–that one is about as good as another as far as nourishment is concerned? But it isn't; one carrot may look and taste like another and yet be lacking in the particular mineral element which our system requires and which carrots are supposed to contain. Laboratory tests prove that the fruits, the vegetables, the grains, the eggs and even the milk and the meats of today are not what they were a few generations ago. (Which doubtless explains why our forefathers [and foremothers] thrived on a selection of foods that would starve us!) No one of today can eat enough fruits and vegetables to supply their system with the mineral salts they require for perfect health, because their stomach isn't big enough to hold them! And we are running to big stomachs.

No longer does a balanced and fully nourishing diet consist merely of so many calories or certain vitamins or a fixed proportion of starches, proteins, and carbohydrates. We now know that it must contain, in addition, something like a score of mineral salts.

It is bad news to learn from our leading authorities that 99 percent of the American people are deficient in these minerals, and that a marked deficiency in any one of the more important minerals actually results in disease. Any upset of the balance, any considerable lack of one or another element, however microscopic the body requirement may be, and we sicken, suffer, shorten our lives.

This discovery is one of the latest and most important contributions of science to the problem of human health.

So far as the records go, the first man in this field of research, the first to demonstrate that most human foods of our day are poor in minerals and that their proportions are not balanced, was Dr. Charles Northen an Alabama physician now living in Orlando, Florida. His discoveries and achievements are of enormous importance to mankind.

Following a wide experience in general practice, Dr. Northen specialized in stomach diseases and nutritional disorder. Later, he moved to New York and made extensive studies along this line, in conjunction with a famous French scientist from Sorbonne. In the course of that work he convinced himself that there was little authentic, definite information on the chemistry of foods, and that no dependence could be placed on existing data.

He asked himself how foods could be used intelligently in the treatment of disease, when they differed so widely in content. The answer seemed to be that they could not be used intelligently. In establishing the fact that serious deficiencies existed and in searching out the reasons therefor, he made an extensive study of the soil. It was he who first voiced the surprising assertion that we must make soil building the basis of food building in order to accomplish human building.

"Bear in mind," says Dr. Northen, "that minerals are vital to human metabolism and health–and that no plant or animal can appropriate to itself any mineral which is not present in the soil upon which it feeds.

"When I first made this statement I was ridiculed, for up to that time people had paid little attention to food deficiencies and even less to soil deficiencies. Men eminent in medicine denied there was any such thing as vegetables and fruits that did not contain sufficient minerals for human needs. Eminent agricultural authorities insisted that all soil contained all necessary minerals. They reasoned that plants take what they need, and that it is the function of the human body to appropriate what it requires. Failure to do so, they said, was a symptom of disorder.

"Some of our respected authorities even claimed that the so-called secondary minerals played no part whatever in human health. It is only recently that such men as Dr. McCollum of Johns Hopkins, Dr. Mendel of Yale, Dr. Sherman of Columbia, Dr. Lipman of Rutgers, and Drs. H.G. Knight and Oswald Schreiner of the United States Department of Agriculture have agreed that these minerals are essential to plant, animal, and human feeding.

"We know that vitamins are complex substances which are indispensable to nutrition, and that each of them is of importance for the normal function of some special structure in the body. Disorder and disease result from any vitamin deficiency.

"It is not commonly realized, however, that vitamins control the body's appropriation of minerals, and in the absence of minerals they have no function to perform. Lacking vitamins, the system can make some use of minerals, but lacking minerals, vitamins are useless.

"Neither does the layman realize that there may be a pronounced difference in both foods and soils–to them one vegetable, one glass of milk, or one egg is about the same as another.

181

Dirt is dirt, too, and they assume that by adding a little fertilizer to it, a satisfactory vegetable or fruit can be grown.

"The truth is that our foods vary enormously in value, and some of them aren't worth eating, as food. For example, vegetation grown in one part of the country may assay 1,100 parts, per billion, of iodine, as against 20 in that grown elsewhere. Processed milk has run anywhere from 362 parts, per million, of iodine and 127 of iron, down to nothing.

"Some of or lands, even unhappily for us, we have been systematically robbing the poor soils and the good soils alike of the very substances most necessary to health, growth, long life, and resistance to disease. Up to the time I began experimenting, almost nothing had been done to make good the theft.

"The more I studied nutritional problems and the effects of mineral deficiencies upon disease, the more plainly I saw that here lay the most direct approach to better health, and the more important it became in my mind to find a method of restoring those missing minerals to our foods.

"The subject interested me so profoundly that I retired from active medical practice and for a good many years now I have devoted myself to it. It's a fascinating subject, for it goes to the heart of human betterment."

The results obtained by Dr. Northen are outstanding. By putting back into foods the stuff that foods are made of, he has proved himself to be a real miracle man of medicine, for he has opened up the shortest and most rational route to better health.

He showed first that it should be done, and then that it could be done. He doubled and redoubled the natural mineral content of fruits and vegetables. He improved the quality of milk by increasing the iron and the iodine in it. He caused hens to lay eggs richer in the vital elements.

By scientific soil feeding, he raised better seed potatoes in Maine, better grapes in California, Better oranges in Florida, and better field crops in other States. (By "better" is meant not only an improvement in food value but also an increase in quantity and quality.)

Before going further into the results he has obtained, let's see just what is involved in this matter of "mineral deficiencies", what it may mean to our health, and how it may effect the growth and development, both mental and physical, of our children.

We know that rats, guinea pigs, and other animals can be fed into a diseased condition and out again by controlling only the minerals in their food.

A 10-year test with rats proved that by withholding calcium they can be bred down to a third the size of those fed with an adequate amount of that mineral. Their intelligence, too, can be controlled by mineral feeding as readily as can their size, their bony structure, and their general health.

Place a number of these little animals inside a maze after starving some of them in a certain mineral element. The starved ones will be unable to find their way out, whereas the others will have little or no difficulty in getting out. Their dispositions can be altered by mineral feeding. They can be made quarrelsome and belligerent; they can even be turned into cannibals and be made to devour each other.

A cage full of normal rats will live in amity. Restrict their calcium, and they will become irritable and draw apart from one another. Then they will begin to fight. Restore their calcium balance and they will grow more friendly; in time they will begin to sleep in a pile as before.

Many backward children are "stupid" merely because they are deficient in magnesia. We punish them for OUR failure to feed them properly.

Certainly our physical well-being is more directly dependent upon the minerals we take into our systems than upon the calories or vitamins or upon the precise proportions of starch, protein, or carbohydrates we consume.

It is now agreed that at least 16 mineral elements are indispensable for normal nutrition, and several more are always found in small amounts in the body, although their precise physiological role has not been determined. Of the 11 indispensable salts, calcium, phosphorous, and iron are perhaps the most important.

Calcium is the dominant nerve controller; it powerfully affects the cell formation of all living things and regulates nerve action. It governs contractability of the muscles and the rhythmic beat of the heart. It also coordinates the other mineral elements and corrects disturbances made by them. It works only in sunlight. Vitamin D is its buddy.

Dr. Sherman of Columbia asserts that 50 percent of the American people are starving for calcium. A recent article in the Journal of the American Medical Association stated that out of 4,000 cases in New York Hospital, only 2 were not suffering from a lack of calcium.

What does such a deficiency mean? How would it affect your health or mine? So many morbid conditions and actual diseases may result that it is almost hopeless to catalog them. Included in the list are rickets, bony deformities, bad teeth, nervous disorders, reduced resistance to other diseases, fatigability, and behavior disturbances such as incorrigibility, assaultiveness, nonadaptability.

Here's one specific example: The soil around a certain Midwest city is poor in calcium. Three hundred children of this community were examined and nearly 90 percent and bad teeth, 69 percent showed affections of the nose and throat, swollen glands, enlarged or diseased tonsils. More than one-third had defective vision, round shoulders, bow legs, and anemia.

Calcium and phosphorous appear to pull in double harness. A child requires as much per day as two grown men, but studies indicate a common deficiency of both in our food. Researches on farm animals point to a deficiency of one or the other as the cause of serious losses to the farmers, and when the soil is poor in phosphorous these animals become bone-chewers. Dr. McCollum says that when there are enough phosphates in the blood there can be no dental decay.

Iron is an essential constituent of the oxygen-carrying pigment of the blood: iron starvation results in anemia, and yet iron cannot be assimilated unless some copper is contained in the diet. In Florida many cattle die from an obscure disease called "salt sickness." It has been found to arise from a lack of iron and copper in the soil and hence in the grass. A man may starve for want of these elements just as a beef "critter" starves.

If Iodine is not present in our foods the function of the thyroid gland is disturbed and goiter afflicts us. The human body requires only fourteen-thousandths of a milligram daily, yet we have a distinct "goiter belt" in the Great Lakes section, and in parts of the Northwest the soil is so poor in iodine that the disease is common.

So it goes, down through the list, each mineral element playing a definite role in nutrition. A characteristic set of symptoms, just as specific as any vitamin-deficiency disease, follows a deficiency in any one of them. It is alarming, therefore, to face the fact that we are starving for these precious, health-giving substances.

Very well, you say, if our foods are poor in the mineral salts they are supposed to contain, why not resort to dosing?

That is precisely what is being done, or attempted. However, those who should know assert that the human system cannot appropriate those elements to the best advantage in any but the food form. At best, only a part of them in the form of drugs can be utilized by the body, and certain dieticians go so far as to say it is a waste of effort to fool with them. Calcium, for instance, cannot be supplied in any form of medication with lasting effect.

But there is a more potent reason why the curing of diet deficiencies by drugging hasn't worked out so well. Consider those 16 indispensable elements and those others which presumably perform some obscure function as yet undetermined. Aside from calcium and phosphorous, they are needed only in infinitesimal quantities, and the activity of one may be dependent upon the presence of another. To determine the precise requirements of each individual case and to attempt to weigh it out on a druggist's scale would appear hopeless.

It is a problem and a serious one. But here is the hopeful side of the picture: Nature can and will solve it if she is encouraged to do so. The minerals in fruit and vegetables are colloidal; i.e. they are in a state of such extremely fine suspension that they can be assimilated by the human system: It is merely a question of giving back to nature the materials with which she works.

We must rebuild our soils: Put back the minerals we have taken out. That sounds difficult but it isn't. Neither is it expensive. Therein lies the short cut to better health and longer life.

When Dr. Northen first asserted that many foods were lacking in mineral content and that this deficiency was due solely to an absence of those elements in the soil, his findings were challenged and he was called a crank. But differences of opinion in the medical profession are not uncommon–it was only 60 years ago that the Medical Society of Boston passed a resolution condemning the use of bathtubs — and he persisted in his assertions that inasmuch as foods did not contain what they were supposed to contain, no physician could with certainty prescribe a diet to overcome physical ills.

He showed that the textbooks are not dependable because many of the analyses in them were made many years ago, perhaps from products raised in virgin soils, whereas our soils have been constantly depleted. Soil analysis, he pointed out, reflect only the content of samples. One analysis may be entirely different from another made 10 miles away.

"And so what?" came the query.

Dr. Northen undertook to demonstrate that something could be done about it. By reestablishing a proper soil balance be actually grew crops that contained an ample amount of desired minerals.

This was incredible. It was contrary to the books and it upset everything connected with diet practice. The scoffers began to pay attention to him. Recently the Southern Medical Association, realizing the hopelessness of trying to remedy nutritional deficiencies without positive factors to work with, recommended a careful study to determine the real mineral content of foodstuffs and the variations due to soil depletion in different localities. These progressive medical men are awake to the importance of prevention.

Dr. Northen went even further and proved that crops grown in a properly mineralized soil were bigger and better; that seeds germinated quicker, grew more rapidly and made larger plants; that trees were healthier and put on more fruit of better quality.

By increasing the mineral content of citrus fruit he likewise improved its texture, its appearance and its flavor.

He experimented with a variety of growing things, and in every case the story was the same. By mineralizing the feed at poultry farms, he got more and better eggs; by balancing pasture soils, he produced richer milk. Persistently he hammered home to farmers, to doctors, and to the general public the thought that life depends upon the minerals.

His work led him into a careful study of the effects of climate, sunlight, ultraviolet and thermal rays upon plant, animal, and human hygiene. In consequence he moved to Florida. People familiar with his work consider him the most valuable man in the State. I met him by reason of the fact that I was harassed by certain soil problems on my Florida farm which had baffled the best chemists and fertilizer experts available.

He is an elderly, retiring man, with a warm smile and an engaging personality, He is a trifle shy until he opens up on his pet topic; then his diffidence disappears and he speaks with authority.

His mind is a storehouse crammed with precise, scientific data about soil, and food chemistry, the complicated life processes of plants, animals, and human beings — and the effect of malnutrition upon all three. He is perhaps as close to the secret of life as any man anywhere.

"Do you call yourself a soil or a food chemist?" I inquired.

"Neither. I'm an M.D. My work lies in the field of biochemistry and nutrition. I gave up medicine because this is a wider and more important work. Sick soils mean sick plants, sick animals, and sick people. Physical, mental, and moral fitness depends largely upon an ample supply and a proper proportion of the minerals in our foods. Nerve function, nerve stability, nerve-cell-building likewise depend thereon. I'm really a doctor of sick soils."

"Do you mean to imply that the vegetables I'm raising on my farm are sick?" I asked.

"Precisely! They're as weak and undernourished as anemic children. They're not much good as food. Look at the pests and the disease that plague them. Insecticides cost farmers nearly as much as fertilizers these days.

"A healthy plant, however, grown in soil properly balanced, can and will resist most insect pests. That very characteristic makes it a better food product. You have tuberculosis and pneumonia germ in your system but you're strong enough to throw them off. Similarly, a really healthy plant will pretty nearly take care of itself in the battle against insects and blights –and will also give the human system what it requires."

"Good heavens! Do you realize what that means to agriculture?"

"Perfectly. Enormous saving. Better crops. Lowered living costs to the rest of us. But I'm not so much interested in agriculture as in health."

"It sounds beautifully theoretical and utterly impractical to me," I told the doctor, whereupon he gave me some of his case records.

For instance, in an orange grove infested with scale, when he restored the mineral balance to part of the soil, the trees growing in that part became clean while the rest remained diseased. By the same means he had grown healthy rosebushes between rows that were riddled by insects.

He had grown tomato and cucumber plants, both healthy and diseased, where the vines intertwined. The bugs ate up the diseased and refused to touch the healthy plants! He showed me interesting analysis of citrus fruit, the chemistry and the food value of which accurately reflected the soil treatment the trees had received.

There is no space here to go fully into Dr. Northen's work but it is of such importance as to rank with that of Burbank, the plant wizard, and with that of our famous physiologists and nutritional experts.

"Healthy plants mean healthy people", said he. "We can't raise a strong race on a weak soil. Why don't you try mending the deficiencies on your farm and growing more minerals into your crops?"

I did try and I succeeded. I was planting a large acreage of celery and under Dr. Northen's direction I fed minerals into certain blocks of the land in varying amounts. When the plants from this soil were mature I had them analyzed, along with celery from other parts of the State. It was the most careful and comprehensive study of the kind ever made, and it included over 250 separate chemical determinations. I was amazed to learn that my celery had more than twice the mineral content of the best grown elsewhere. Furthermore, it kept much better, with and without refrigeration, proving that the cell structure was sounder.

In 1927, Mr. W. W. Kincaid, a "gentleman farmer" of Niagara Falls, heard an address by Dr. Northen and was so impressed that he began extensive experiments in the mineral feeding of plants and animals. The results he has accomplished are conspicuous. He set himself the task of increasing the iodine in the milk from his dairy herd. He has succeeded in adding both iodine and iron so liberally that one glass of his milk contains all of these minerals that an adult person requires for a day.

Is this significant? Listen to these incredible figures taken from a bulletin of the South Carolina Food Research Commission: "In many sections three out of five persons have goiter and a recent estimate states that 30 million people in the United States suffer from it."

Foods rich in iodine are of the greatest importance to these sufferers.

Mr Kincaid took a brown Swiss heifer calf which was dropped in the stockyards, and by raising her on mineralized pasturage and a properly balanced diet made her the third all-time champion of her breed! In one season she gave 21,924 pounds of milk. He raised her butterfat production from 410 pounds in 1 year to 1,037 pounds. Results like these are of incalculable importance.

Others besides Mr. Kincaid are following the trail Dr. Northen blazed. Similar experiments with milk have been made in Illinois and nearly every fertilizer company is beginning to urge use of the rare mineral elements. As an example I quote from statements of a subsidiary of one of the leading copper companies:

Many States show a marked reduction in the productive capacity of the soil * * * in many districts amounting to a 25 to 50 percent reduction in the last 50 years * * *. Some areas show a tenfold variation in calcium. Some show a sixtyfold variation in phosphorus * * *. Authorities * * * see soil depletion, barren livestock, increased human death rate due to heart disease, deformities, arthritis, increased dental caries, all due to lack of essential minerals in plant food.

"It is neither a complicated nor an expensive undertaking to restore our soils to balance and thereby work a real miracle in the control of disease," says Dr. Northen. "As a matter of fact, it's a money-making move for the farmer, and any competent soil chemist can tell them how to proceed.

"First determine by analysis the precise chemistry of any given soil, then correct the deficiencies by putting down enough of the missing elements to restore its balance. The same care should be used as in prescribing for a sick patient, for proportions are of vital importance.

"In my early experiments I found it extremely difficult to get the variety of minerals needed in the form in which I wanted to use them but advancement in chemistry, and especially our ever-increasing knowledge of colloidal chemistry, has solved that difficulty. It is now possible, by use of minerals in colloidal form, to prescribe a cheap and effective system of soil correction which meets this vital need and one which fits in admirably with nature's plans.

"Soils seriously deficient in minerals cannot produce plant life competent to maintain our needs, and with the continuous cropping and shipping away of those concentrates, the condition becomes worse.

———

"A famous nutrition authority recently said, 'One sure way to end the American people's susceptibility to infection is to supply through food a balanced ration of iron, copper, and other metals. An organism supplied with a diet adequate to, or preferably in excess of, all mineral requirements may so utilize these elements as to produce artificially by our present method of immunization. You can't make up the deficiency by using patent medicine.'

"He's absolutely right. Prevention of disease is easier, more practical, and more economical than cure, but not until foods are standardized on a basis of what they contain instead of what they look like can the dietician prescribe them with intelligence and with effect.

"There was a time when medical therapy had no standards because the therapeutic elements in drugs had not been definitely determined on a chemical basis. Pharmaceutical houses have changed all that. Food chemistry, on the other hand, has depended almost entirely upon governmental agencies for its research, and in our real knowledge of values we are about where medicine was a century ago.

"Disease preys most surely and most viciously on the undernourishment and unfit plants, animals, and human beings alike, and when the importance of these obscure mineral elements is fully realized the chemistry of life will have to be rewritten. No one knows their mental or bodily capacity, how well they can feel or how long they can live, for we are all cripples and weaklings. It is a disgrace to science. Happily, that chemistry is being rewritten and we are on our way to better health by returning to the soil the things we have stolen from it.

"The public can help; it can hasten the change. How? By demanding quality in its food. By insisting that our doctors and our health departments establish scientific standards of nutritional value.

"The growers will quickly respond. They can put back those minerals almost overnight, and by doing so they can actually make money through bigger and better crops.

"It is simpler to cure sick soils than sick people — which shall we choose?"

www.betterhealththruresearch.com/US SenateDocument.htm
bioelectrichelth.org/MMM 1936.htm

Glossary

A

ACE inhibitors—angiotensin-converting enzyme inhibitor; pharmaceutical drug used primarily to try to control hypertension.

Acetylcholine—one of the major stimulatory neurotransmitters.

Alpha lipoic acid—an antioxidant. Yeast, liver, kidney, spinach, broccoli, and potatoes are good sources of alpha-lipoic acid. It has the ability to recycle other anti-oxidants like Vitamins C and E. It helps convert carbohydrates into energy in the mitochondria.

Alzheimer's—the most common form of dementia; the fastest growing cause of death in the US.

Amyloid plaques—a characteristic degenerative change in the brains of Alzheimer patients.

Androstenedione—an intermediary hormone manufactured in the adrenal cortex formed from DHEA or progesterone that can become testosterone or estrone.

Angiotensin—a hormone that causes vasoconstriction and increased blood pressure.

Anxiety—a feeling of fear, uneasiness, or worry about something in the future.

Asparagine—a non-essential amino acid used in the synthesis of brain or nerve cells.

Asthma—a reoccurring illness involving the respiratory passages that are thought to be caused by a combination of genetic variances and food/chemical allergy/sensitivity (avoid Tylenol products).

ATP—adenosine triphosphate; the cellular fuel of the mitochondria from glucose.

B

B1—thiamine.

B2—riboflavin.

B3—niacin; lowers LDLs and triglycerides and increases HDLs; important for liver detoxification; vasodilator.

B4—adenine.

B5—pantothenic acid; important for adrenal health.

B6—pyridoxine.

B7—biotin.

B8—inositol.

B9—folic acid.

B10—PABA/para-aminobenzoic acid.

B11—salicylic acid.

B12—cobalamin. Use methylated forms like methylcobolamine vs. cynacobolamine.

Bariatric surgery—a surgical procedure that involves reducing the size of the stomach causing major absorption problems of key nutrients.

Biotin—Vitamin B7.

Breast Cancer—cancer involving the breast tissue that can be related to excess carcinogenic estrogen metabolites; risk can be reduced by appropriate micronutrient intake.

C

Calcium—one of the major minerals in the body, especially the bone.

Carnitine—an amino acid that is important in the transport of fatty acids into the mitochondrial energy production in the cells.

Celiac Disease—a chronic inflammation of the small intestine due to an allergy to wheat proteins; can cause auto-immune responses, leaky gut, and many nutritional deficiencies due to malabsorption.

Ceruloplasmin—a major copper-carrying protein involved with iron absorption.

Calcium –D- glutarate—nutrient that positively influences the microbiome in reducing a substance that increase certain cancer risks, helps in estrogen detoxification, and lipid lowering.

Cholesterol—a substance produced by the liver that acts as a carrier of fats and is the source for all the sex hormones, glucocorticoids, mineralocorticoids, and Vitamin D.

Choline—water soluble nutrient often classified as a B Vitamin that is involved in methylation processes and cell membrane functions; reduces a fatty liver.

Chromium—a micronutrient that is essential in insulin/glucose regulation.

CoenzymeQ10—an anti-oxidant necessary in cell energy production that decreases in the aging process and is depleted by statin medications.

Cognitive—concerned with the act or process of understanding, knowing, or perceiving.

Colitis—inflammation of the colon, often due to auto-immune response.

COMT—catechol-o-methyl-transferase; an enzyme involved in estrogen detoxification that has gene variants that require 300-400% increase in methylating B Vitamins, such as folic acid, B6, and B12 for normal function to take place.

Copper—a trace mineral that can be depleted by excess zinc supplementation; deficiency associated with degenerative neurological conditions.

Corticosteroid—consists of two types of two types of hormones produced by the adrenal cortex- the glucosteroids and the mineralocorticoids.

Cortisol—one of the primary glucosteroids produced in the adrenal cortex that is involved in activating glucose for energy needs and is a powerful anti-inflammatory for the body.

Cysteine—a sulfur containing amino acid that is the limiting factor in glutathione production used in many liver detoxification processes.

Cytokines—regulatory messengers involved in inflammatory processes.

D

Depression—a feeling of sadness and disinterest in life; some 19 million Americans are medicated for this.

DHA—(docosahexaenoic acid); an omega 3 fatty acid that is the major structural component of the brain, skin, sperm, and retina.

DHEA—(dehydroepiandrosterone); a hormone that is produced from pregnenolone and becomes testosterone or estrone through the intermediary, androstenedione.

Diabetes—three types- Type 1 involves pancreatic beta cell failure at an early age; Type 2 usually involves a metabolic dysfunction denoted by obesity and insulin resistance; Type 3 usually involves pancreatic beta cell failure later in life concomitant with earlier insulin resistance.

DNA—(deoxyribonucleic acid), is the hereditary material in humans.

Dopamine—one of the primary stimulatory neurotransmitters and is located in the frontal brain. Most addictive substances such as sugar, alcohol, and cocaine stimulate dopamine. A deficiency in the substantia nigra is associated with Parkinson's.

Dyslipidemia—an imbalance in HDL cholesterol, LDL cholesterol, and/or triglycerides.

E

Endometrium—the mucous membrane in the uterus that thickens under the influence of estrogen in the first fourteen days of the menstrual cycle in preparation of implantation. Thickening often occurs during perimenopause due to a progesterone deficiency.

Endothelin—a peptide that is a powerful vasoconstrictor that is produced by the vascular endothelium.

EPA—(eicosapentaenoic acid); an omega 3 fatty acid that is associated with many health benefits in fetal development, brain, and cardiovascular health and inflammatory ructions.

Epinephrine—(adrenaline); a chemical produced in the adrenal medulla that is activated in a fight/flight response.

Estradiol—(E2); the dominant hormone in women during child-bearing years; 12x more powerful than estrone and 80x more powerful than estriol; balanced by progesterone.

Estriol—(E3); the benign form of estrogen; end of the sex hormone cascade; important to reduce hot flashes, vaginal dryness, and insomnia in peri- and menopausal women.

Estrogen—the largest hormone pool in younger women consisting of estrone, estradiol, and estriol.

F

Fatigue—feeling weak, constantly tired, lack of energy; multiple causes including low thyroid, low adrenal, anemia, heart dysfunction, mitochondrial energy utilization.

Fertility—the natural ability to produce offspring. Currently 15 % of American couples cannot reproduce. Most of the causes are due to micronutrient deficiencies coupled with excess body burden of environmental endocrine disruptors.

Fibromyalgia—a medical condition causes by mitochondrial dysfunction in the muscles; usually involves low thyroid and adrenal function, Vitamin D deficiency, and multiple micronutrient deficiencies involving the mitochondrial energy production.

Folate—the natural form of the B9 Vitamin found in abundance in deep green leafy vegetables. Forty to seventy percent of the population has a gene variant involving folate often necessitating supplementation.

Folic acid—the supplemented form of folate, often in synthetic form vs. natural form.

Follicles—a fluid filled sac in the ovaries that produces an egg.
Fructose intolerance—a fairly common metabolic problem with breaking down fructose. Unlike other sugars, fructose can only be broken down in the liver. People with this should avoid fruit juices and especially high fructose corn syrup. High fructose corn syrup is neurotoxin and disrupts the function of the hormone, leptin, which satisfies our appetite.

G

GABA—(gamma-aminobutyric acid); one of the two primary inhibitory neurotransmitters in the brain. Fifty percent of the world's population is GABA dominant.
Glutamine—an amino acid that is found in abundance in the skeletal muscle and is important in stomach and small intestine health.
Glutathione—one of the most powerful antioxidants in the body; helps recycle other antioxidants; especially important in numerous liver detoxification processes.
Glutathione peroxidase—an antioxidant enzyme crucial for scavenging free radicals in the body involving hydrogen and lipids; protects the cell membranes.
GPx—abbreviation for glutathione peroxidase.

H

HbA1C—(glycated hemoglobin); indicates the 60 day average of blood sugars.
HCL—hydrochloric acid produced in the stomach.
HDL—(high density lipoproteins); larger carriers of cholesterol; HDL2b is the most efficient cleaner of LDLs back to the liver.
Headaches—pain anywhere in the head; multiple types – tension headaches, migraines more common in women related to food/chemical allergy/sensitivity or estrogen dominance during menstrual cycle, cluster headaches more common in men.
Histamine—a substance involved in allergic reactions that cause blood vessels to become dilated and more permeable; contained in some foods that should be restricted in susceptible individuals.
H-P-A axis—(hypothalamus-pituitary-adrenal axis); the mechanism that controls the hormone production in the adrenal glands.
HRT—(hormone replacement therapy); usually refers to the synthetic form.

Hypertension—elevated blood pressure, currently defined as systolic pressure above 140 and/or diastolic pressure above 90.
Hypothyroidism—an under function of the thyroid; a common problem in America of epidemic proportions, especially in menopausal women; under diagnosed due to too broad normal reference ranges and thyroid receptor resistance.

I

Inflammation—a complex biological response involving the white blood cells to a chemical or mechanical or emotional stressor; all chronic disease involves an excess of inflammation.
Inositol—(B8); important in brain functions and helps prevent, reduce fatty liver from excess sugar intake.
Insomnia—difficulty falling asleep or staying asleep; can involve micronutrient deficiencies, neurotransmitter or hormonal imbalances, liver dysfunction.
Insulin resistance—when there is adequate insulin production but there is cell receptor resistance to accepting the insulin into the cell, which causes serum blood sugar levels to be higher and mitochondrial energy production lower.
IVF—in vitro fertility.

L

L–carnitine—synthesized from the amino acids lysine and methionine; important nutrient in the introduction of fatty acids into the mitochondrial energy chain of the cell.
LDL—(low density lipoprotein); smaller carriers for cholesterol that can increases the potential of damage to the blood vessel wall if the endothelium is not healthy.
Lipoprotein A—a sticky, VLDL that is inherited and increases cardiovascular risks but is negated by adequate amounts of specific micronutrients such as Vitamin C, B Vitamins, lysine, and proline.

M

Magnesium—a major mineral in the body; 80 % of Americans are deficient without supplementation.
Malabsorption—inadequate digestion of proteins, fats, or carbohydrates due to lack of hydrochloric acid production in the stomach, reduced pancreatic enzymes production, reduce bile production or gall bladder surgery, small intestine dysfunction.

Manganese—a trace mineral, especially important for tendon, ligament repair.

Melatonin—the oldest hormone that is in all plants and animals; the most powerful anti-oxidant the body produces; involved with sleep/wake cycle; no negative feedback system associated with supplementation.

Menopause—when a women has not had a menstrual cycle for 1 year denoted by a significant reduction in most sex hormones including progesterone, estrogen, DHEA, and testosterone.

Methylation—the process whereby a CH3+ molecule is added to a substance; an essential process in most detoxification pathways.

Migraine—a type of vascular-related headache more common to women, usually related to food/chemical allergy/sensitivity or estrogen dominance in menstrual cycle.

Miscarriage—the spontaneous abortion of the fetus before it can live independently; can be related to genetic problems, nutritional/ hormonal deficiencies, or excess environmental toxins in the mother.

Mitochondria—the power plant within each cell that makes energy for the body.

MTHFR—a common gene variant involving folate absorption, necessitating a greater intake of this critical B Vitamin.

Myelin sheath—a fatty substance consisting of a great deal of cholesterol that surrounds and insulates the axon nerves.

Myopathy—a condition, such as statin medications, that can cause muscle destruction.

N

N–acetyl–cysteine—a precursor for glutathione.

Neurotransmitters—chemical/electrical messengers that transfer information from one nerve to another at the synapse.

Niacin—Vitamin B3.

NMDA—N-methyl-D-aspartate; a specific type of brain receptor that is especially susceptible to excitotoxins from MSG and aspartame that can lead to brain cell death.

O

Obesity—an overweight condition that increases risk of many diseases and early death; usually considered if BMI is over 30.

Omega 3 fatty acids—essential polyunsaturated fatty acids that come from food sources that are necessary for optimum health.

Omega 6 fatty acids—essential polyunsaturated fatty acids that come in anti-inflammatory and pro-inflammatory forms; hydrogenated and trans-fats are pro-inflammatory.

Osteoblast—a cell from fibroblasts that make a new bone cell.

Osteoclast—a cell that is responsible for bone resorption; prescription drugs are designed to inhibit these cells but do nothing to stimulate new bone cell growth.

Osteoporosis—a loss of bone density resulting from a loss of tensile strength more so than a loss of calcium.

P

Pain—physical discomfort caused by illness and injury; a growing problem in our society due to excess weight causing inflammation.

Pantothenate—Vitamin B5.

Pantothenic acid—the water soluble B5 that is important in the processes of protein, fat, and carbohydrate breakdown, multiple enzymes involved in brain and central nervous system communication, and adrenal function.

PCOS—polycystic ovary syndrome); a metabolic syndrome combination of adrenal hyperfunction causing excess cortisol and glucose production and lack of conversion of testosterone to estrogen.

Pellagra—severe niacin deficiency.

PH—a measurement of hydrogen ion concentration from 0-14 with 7 being neutral. Measurements under 7 are considered acidic while measurements over 7 are considered alkaline or basic.

Phosphotidylserine—an important phospholipid component of all cell membranes.

PMS—(pre-menstrual syndrome); symptoms such as water retention, cramping, anxiousness, nervousness, and irritability before the beginning of the menstrual cycle caused by an imbalance between estrogen and progesterone, usually because of a relative or true progesterone deficiency.

Pregnancy—the time when one or more offspring develop inside a woman.

Pregnenolone—the first sex hormone produced from cholesterol in the adrenal cortex. It becomes DHEA in one pathway and progesterone in the other.

Progesterone—the balancing antagonist to estradiol that is dominant after ovulation and throughout pregnancy.

Prolactin—a hormone produced by the pituitary that enables women to produce milk.

R
Riboflavin—B1.
Ritalin—a commonly prescribed medication for hyperactivity in children.

S
SAMe—(s-adenosyl-methionine); a substance that is made from an interaction between methionine and adenosine triphosphate; a methyl donor in many crucial enzyme activities.
Selenium—a trace mineral essential in the conversion of T4 into T3 in the liver.
Selenoproteins—members of a protein family that all contain selenium and many common cofactors that are involved in a variety of processes including cardiovascular and immune health.
Serine—a non-essential protein derived from glycine; deficiencies could indicate genetic variances in enzymes that convert and have been associated with neuropathies and neuritis; important component of phosphotidylserine, an integral component of all cell membranes.
Serotonin—an inhibitory neurotransmitter associated with a sense of well-being that is produced by sun light striking the eyes. It is converted into melatonin.
Sleep apnea—a sleep disorder associated with breathing interruptions.
Spectrox^T—the cumulative anti-oxidant capabilities in the spectracell test.
Superoxide dismutase—a powerful anti-oxidant the body produces to protect the mitochondria and the mitochondrial membrane.
Synaptic plasticity—the ability of the synapses to increase and expand or decrease and shrink based on activity or reinforcement.

T
T3—(triiodothyronine); the more bio-active form of thyroid hormone produced in the liver from T4.
T4—(thyroxine); produced in the thyroid from TSH thyroid stimulating hormone from the pituitary, dependent upon adequate iodine.

Telomeres—a region at the end of the chromosome that protects it from deterioration.

Testosterone—the androgenic hormone produced from DHEA or progesterone.

Thiamine—Vitamin B1.

TNF-a—(tumor necrosis factor-alpha); increases when the bod is fighting an infection or cancer; can be triggered in auto-immune diseases as well.

Triglycerides—a type of fat produced by the liver from excess sugar, especially fructose.

Tryptophan—an essential amino acid that converts into serotonin and niacin if it has necessary co-factors.

TSH—(thyroid-stimulating hormone); a stimulating hormone produced by the pituitary that signals the thyroid to produce thyroxine (T4).

V

Vitamin A—a fat soluble vitamin that comes from two sources – pre-formed retinoids found in kidney, liver, and eggs and carotenoids in dark green, yellow, or orange vegetables; necessary for mitochondrial energy production and important in skin, eye, and immune health.

Vitamin C—a water and oil soluble vitamin that humans do not produce; essential in blood vessel integrity and collagen repair and immune response.

Vitamin D—a fat soluble vitamin/hormone that is derived from cholesterol and stimulated by sun light on the skin; increases intestinal absorption of calcium, magnesium, phosphate, and zinc; deficiency under 19.6 ng/mL is associated with all disease morbidity.

Vitamin E—a fat soluble vitamin found in nuts, seeds, and deep green leafy vegetables; anti-oxidant for lipid peroxidation occurring in the cell membranes.

W

Weight management—strategy for maintaining optimum weight for health.

Z

Zinc—an important trace mineral in over 300 enzymes in the body. Deficiencies can occur from hypochlorhydria and Vitamin D deficiency. Important in prostate health, immune response, and conversion of T4 to T3.

About the Author

Dr. Kelly Miller is a 1980 graduate of Logan University of Health Sciences in St. Louis, Missouri, receiving his Doctor of Chiropractic degree.

He received a Certification in Industrial/Occupational Health from Northwestern Chiropractic College in 1991.

He worked as an ergonomic, safety-consultant and after-care doctor for Food Barn, Ball's Price Chopper, and Twentieth Century in the Kansas City Metropolitan area in the 1990's.

He received his certificate in Acupuncture in 1996, and is a Fellow of the Acupuncture Society of America.

In 2001, he received his Certification as a Naturopathic Medical Doctor from the National Accreditation and Certification of Naturopathic Medical Doctors in Washington DC.

He finished his Fellowship in Aging and Regenerative Medicine from the Brazil-American Academy of Aging and Regenerative Medicine in San Paulo, Brazil, in March 2014.

He received his Certification in Functional Diagnostic Medicine from Functional Medicine University in December 2014.

Dr. Miller's clinical practice covers over thirty-five years, treating over fifteen thousand patients. He is an international lecturer on the genetic, nutritional, and hormonal considerations related to heart health.

Made in the USA
Las Vegas, NV
20 March 2024

87517079R00125